MW01484069

Quick Reference Guide

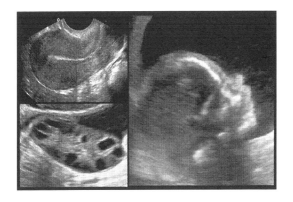

for Ob & Gyn Sonography

NOTICE:

Neither the Publisher nor the Author assumes any responsibility for any loss or injury and/or damage to persons or property arising out of or related to any of the information contained in this book. It is the responsibility of the treating practitioner to determine the treatment and method of application for the patient.

No part of this publication may be reproduced, stored or transmitted in any form or by any means, electronic or otherwise without written permission from the author.

Limitations of this book:

Please note that the information contained in this guide is not intended to be used as a textbook, but is merely an overview of some of the most common findings in ob/gyn sonography. It should only be used after the successful completion of an accredited ultrasound program and will not replace the many comprehensive textbooks available.

This book is dedicated to my husband, Tim, for putting up with my crazy idea to write an ultrasound book, and to my mother, Linda, for telling me I was smart enough to write an ultrasound book.

ACKNOWLEDGMENTS:

I would like to thank the following teachers, doctors and sonographers who contributed to my learning over the years, and those who submitted suggestions they felt would be of help to other sonographers:

Renato M. Augustin, MD, RDMS, RVT
Diane Bernal, RDMS
Chana Bitton-Friedman, BS, RDMS
Jennifer Blaylock, RDMS
Stephen Carlan, MD
Blanca Caro, MD, RDMS, MSCR
Lorena Castillo, RDMS
Cindy Cerverizzo, RDMS, RVT
Franklyn Christensen, MD
Heather Duval-Foote, BAS, RDMS
Armando Fuentes, MD
Vanessa Gonzalez, DMS
Lynn Hurlburt, RDMS
Julia Imboden, MS, RDMS, RVT, RDCS
Kristina Kinnunen, RDMS
Yogan Kisten, DMS
Selma Kurtovic, DMS
James Maher, MD
Ashlea McCauley, RT
Jessica Meyers, DMS

Gwen Miller, RDMS
Kelly Montgomery, RDMS
Miriam Ortiz, DMS
Katie Pan, DMS
Alicia Parker, RDMS
Patricia Phipps, DMS
Tatiana Pinto, RDMS
Erika Pohlad, RDMS
Maria Roman Peralta, RDMS
Julie Sadlier, RDMS
Tara Shedden, DMS
Wendy Sousa, RDMS
Susan Thompson, RDMS RVT
David Toms, MD
Shima Whitehead, DMS
JoAnn Wilcox, RDMS, RT, RVT
Monica Williams, DMS
Richelle Winter, RDMS
Paula Woletz, MPH, RDMS, RDCS
Dwan Wright, RDMS

Charlotte Henningsen, MS, RT, RDMS, RVT, FSDMS
Patty Moraino-Braga MS Ed, RDMS, RVT, RDCS, RT
Melinda Shoen, MSM, RDMS, RVT, RDCS

And many thanks to the doctors of Women's Care Florida, Ob & Gyn Specialists for supporting this project:

N. Donald Diebel, MD, PhD
Arnold Lazar, MD
Mark Wilstrup, MD
Theresa Carducci, MD
Sheryl Logan, MD
Marnique Jones, MD

Denise Durkee, MD
Ann Marie D'Heureux, MD
Sanjay Tandon, MD
Rebecca Weber, MD
Wendy Quirino, MD
George Amyradkis, MD

Preface
(PLEASE READ THIS FIRST)

Before graduating from ultrasound school, I started writing down important things I didn't want to forget in a mini three-ring binder, things like protocols and normal measurements. Once I started my first job, it gave me a little sense of security knowing I had a reference book tucked in my scrub pocket. Over the years, I've added more great information to my notebook, like common abbreviations the doctors use, some Spanish phrases, and words I can never remember how to spell (is it mennorhagia or menorrhagia???). It has become so useful to me that I thought other sonographers would like to have one too, so I decided to write a quick reference guide.

There are many small reference-style books available, but they are all written by physicians and seemed to contain a lot of "filler" information, like the history of the piezoelectric crystal (very interesting, but I don't need that information at my fingertips). This book is different because it was written by a practicing sonographer, with much thought put into what you WILL need at your fingertips.

I've divided the book into two main sections: Gynecology and Obstetrics. Each section contains measurement information, protocols, common findings and a blank page for your own notes.

Pay careful attention to the Key Points pages within the sections. Here you will find important reminders, tips, tricks and pitfalls to avoid. I've also added a few tips for your reports in *"italics."*

In the back, you will find terms and abbreviations, helpful websites, Spanish phrases and a blank page to record contact information (networking!). Most of the diagrams found in the ob and gyn sections are duplicated in the back for you to cut-out and display in a visible spot.

In addition, it will be helpful for you to keep a textbook handy at your desk for more in-depth information. I've listed some of my favorites in the back of this book.

After six months to a year, you will feel more comfortable performing your scans, but keep in mind that although experience is the best teacher, you will never know everything. Even veteran sonographers get cases they can't figure out.

I hope you will find this book helpful and informative. I wish you great success, and may you always have the same desire to learn as you do now!

-RSW

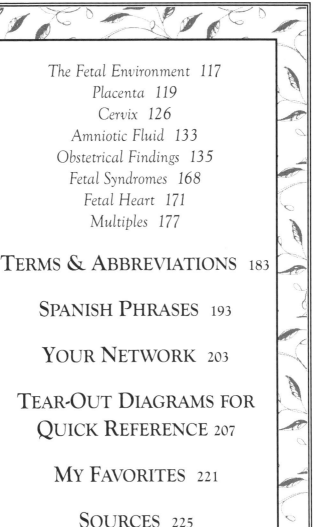

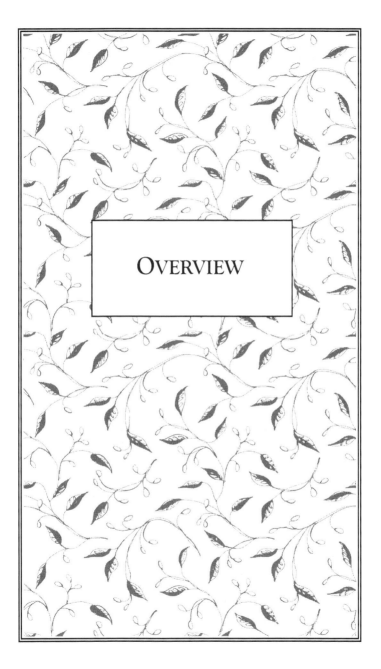

OVERVIEW

KEY POINTS FOR PATIENT CARE AND WORK ENVIRONMENT

- Always greet the patient with a smile and tell them your name, then verify their name and the reason you are performing the exam.

- It's a good idea to state up front that you will not be able to give the results of the exam to the patient: "The doctor will need to review the images, then he will discuss the results with you." This will help prevent them from assuming there is something wrong if you evade their questions.

- Patients want to feel understood, validated and cared about. Be kind and sympathetic, even if you are having a bad day or are running behind schedule. Treat them as if they were a member of your family.

- Keep in mind that the patient is watching your expression and listening to everything you say as you are scanning.

- Being a good sonographer means more than just acquiring good images. It may mean holding the patient's hand, listening to their concerns, even educating the patient on what ultrasound is and what we really do.

- If you need to discuss your findings with the doctor, be sure to have a brief patient history ready in case you are asked for it (patient age, LMP, weeks of gestation, etc.).

- Come to work fully rested and with a good attitude. Do not allow your personal life to interfere with your job performance.

- Smile and say hello to everyone you pass by. Being in a good mood is contagious!

- Every member of the office or hospital plays an important role. Treat everyone with kindness and respect.

- If a coworker makes a mistake that inconveniences you, simply accept their apology and reassure them that we all make mistakes and it is no big deal.

- At times, your manager might ask you do something that is inconvenient for you, such as traveling to another site to fill in for a sick employee. "Sure, no problem," is exactly the response that will gain you favorability and job security.

- Try to avoid office gossip and negativity. Always remember, your **attitude** is just as important as your scanning skills.

- Become registered in at least two modalities. Some employers require it, plus, passing a registry exam earns you 15 CME credits.

- Networking is a great way to hear about new job opportunities. Try to attend as many conferences and seminars as you can. Join local and national ultrasound societies.

Keep learning! Take every opportunity available to learn new information and techniques.

IMAGE ORIENTATION

Transabdominal:

The top of your monitor is the location of the probe; orientation will change with transabdominal or transvaginal scanning. When you are scanning transabdominaly, your transducer is perpendicular to the patient, aiming at the floor. The patient's head is towards the left of your screen and the patient's feet are toward the right.

ANTERIOR

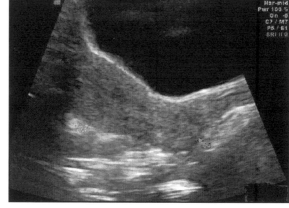

HEAD

FEET

POSTERIOR

Transsvaginal:

When you are scanning transvaginaly, your probe is in the vaginal canal and is now parallel with the patient, aiming at the patient's head. **The orientation of the image on your screen has changed.** Now the patient's head is toward the bottom of the screen and her feet are towards the top of the screen. Turning your transducer transverse is actually giving you a coronal image of the pelvis.

FEET

ANTERIOR

POSTERIOR

HEAD

Ultrasound Physics Analogies

Output Power: If a penny is placed in a glass of water you can look down into the glass and still see the detail in the penny. If you start to tap the side of the glass, vibrations/waves are created causing the details to blur. The harder you tap, the more vibrations you create and the harder it is to see the penny. Ouput power vibrates tissue (Harmonics), so to improve clarity and detail, reduce the overall Output.

Harmonics: Tissues vibrate at twice the frequency from the initial frequency. The higher the frequency, the better the image quality. So if a fetus was insonated at 5 MHz, then the Harmonic frequency would be 10 MHz. The 10 MHz will have better image quality but the negative effect might be limited penetration.

Depth: Changing depth is similar to walking up and down bleacher steps to get closer or further away from the action at a football game.

Read Zoom: Can be performed both pre and post processing; similar to using binoculars; does not improve image quality just magnifies the image.

Write Zoom: Pre processing only. Imagine taking a wallet size photo and enlarging it on a copy machine to an 8 x 10 size. The wallet size image will be sharper because the image is compressed (tighter lines). The 8x10 has same number of lines but is stretched to accommodate the size. Using the zoom ROI box, you are compressing the same number of lines into a smaller box therefore improving image quality and frame rate.

Focus: In a sound wave, there is the same number of scan lines from near field to far field. As the sound wave travels, the beam narrows, tightening the scan lines. This is very similar to an hour glass shape. The image quality is the best at this level due to the compressed scan lines. The focal zone can be moved to the area of interest for the best resolution of a structure.

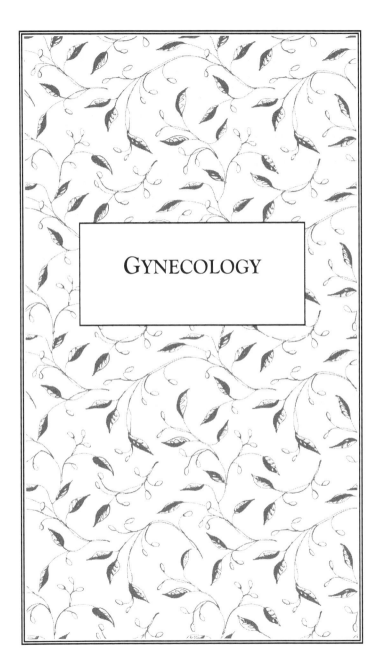

GYNECOLOGY

KEY POINTS FOR GYNECOLOGY

🔑 It is vitally important that you read the patient's history before starting the exam. For example, the patient's age will play a key role in the diagnosis. A 68 year old woman has most likely gone through menopause and will no longer be ovulating, therefore a mass on the ovary would not be diagnosed as a corpus luteal cyst.

🔑 Be sure the patient has a completely EMPTY bladder before you begin a transvaginal exam; urine in the bladder will cause image artifacts.

🔑 Always begin with a left to right sagital sweep and an anterior to posterior transverse sweep of the pelvis. This will minimize the chance of missing an adnexal mass, pedunculated fibroid or congenital anomaly such as a bicornuate uterus.

🔑 It is important to note in your report the amount of cul-de-sac fluid you see. Some sites will require an anterior/posterior measurement, while others will simply have you classify it as mild, moderate or severe. If you see fluid in the anterior cul-de-sac, scan the patient transabdominaly to see how high the fluid goes.

🔑 It may be difficult to know where to place your calipers when measuring a uterus with a large fibroid. It is best to include the fibroid in the measurement if it is clearly within the myometrium. If it is pedunculated, do not include it in your measurement.

If you suspect a uterine fibroid but can't make out the borders, change your image color to sepia and you will more easily see the margins.

If you are having trouble finding the ovaries, angle your probe toward the uterine fundus, turn your probe transverse, then slowly move laterally right or left until you reach the iliac vessel. The ovary will usually be anterior and medial to this vessel, however, the ovaries are often spotted down in the cul-de-sac or posterior to the fundus as well (especially the left ovary). Slowly sweep your probe anterior to posterior until you see the ovary. Applying pressure to the patient's abdomen will help move bowel out of your way. If you have trouble with one side, move to the other. This may give the bowel time to lift from the contra-lateral side.

If you don't find the ovary using these techniques, it may be located more superior in the pelvis; switch to your abdominal probe and search transabdominaly. Move your probe to the opposite side of the pelvis and use the bladder as a window, i.e. scanning from the left and angling towards the right to visualize the right ovary. Adjusting your image contrast may also help.

Be sure to note in your report the method you used to find the ovary, or that you were not able to find it at all: *"Left ovary was seen best transabdominaly; right ovary was not seen due to overlying bowel and gas; attempts were made TV and TA."*

Fallopian tubes aren't usually seen unless they are fluid filled, called hydrosalpinx.

Bowel can have many different appearances. When fluid filled, it will have an anechoic appearance and you may see echogenic matter peristalsing within. Bowel is commonly mistaken for ovaries, adnexal masses and even an edemic uterus. In transverse, bowel will usually have a spokewheel appearance. When in doubt, apply abdominal pressure and watch for peristalsing.

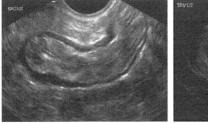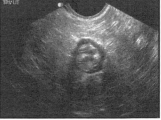

Bowel mistaken for the uterus: The sagital image above shows a loop of bowel resembling a diseased uterus but in transverse, it has the typical spokewheel appearance of bowel.

Adnexal masses vary greatly in size and appearance. It can be difficult to distinguish between a normal, physiological mass, such as a hemorrhagic corpus luteal cyst, and a worrisome mass, such as a granulosum cell tumor because some clues are seen in both benign and malignant lesions. This is why it is important to just report what you see and allow the physician to take it from there. Refer to the Common Pelvic Findings section of this book for more information.

PELVIC ANATOMY MEASUREMENTS

Uterus (L x W x H) average:
Nulliparous: 6 x 4 x 3 cm
Multiparous: 8 x 5 x 4 cm
Postmenopausal: 5 x 4 x 3 cm

Endometrium:
2-15 mm premenopausal
<5 mm postmenopausal
<8 mm on hormone therapy

Ovary (L x W x H) average: 3 x 2 x 2 cm
Ovaries will appear smaller and may be difficult to visualize on a postmenopausal patient.

Remember, these are just AVERAGE measurements; every woman is a little different.

NOTES:

PROTOCOLS FOR GYNECOLOGY

TRANSVAGINAL

Performed with an **EMPTY** bladder.

CVX/CDS
UT SAG
UT TRV
ENDO
RT OV TRV
RT OV SAG
RT ADX
LT OV TRV
LT OV SAG
LT ADX

1. Begin in sagital, slowly entering the vagina. Watch the screen as you go.

2. Image the cervix and cul-de-sac; note any visible nabothian cysts, masses or fluid.

3. Measure the uterus in three dimensions. Images should be made with and without measurements. Image the left and right side of the uterus. If fibroids are visible, measure the three largest and note their locations.

4. Evaluate the endometrium. Measure the anterior to posterior thickness (echogenic stripe to echogenic stripe), and use color Doppler to evaluate its vascularity. Note any visible masses or an IUD if applicable.

5. Measure both ovaries in three dimensions. Measure cysts larger than 2 cm and use color Doppler to evaluate their vascularity.

6. Evaluate the adnexas. Measure any masses and note any fluid collections.

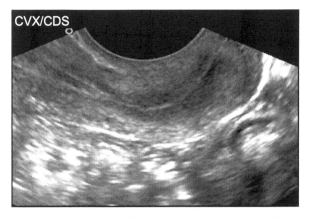

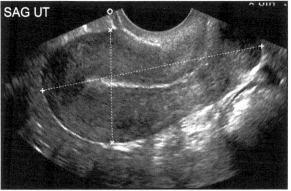

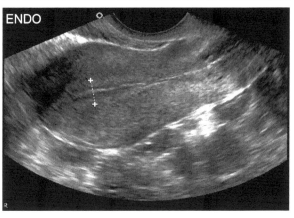

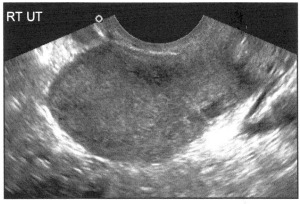

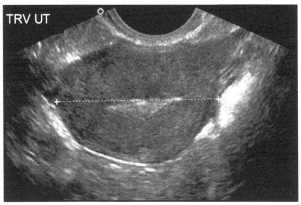

24

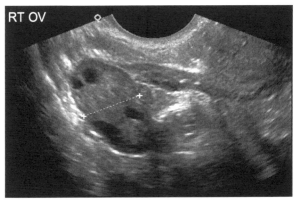

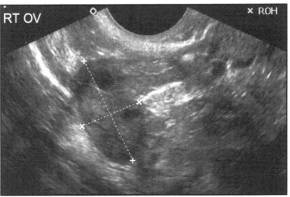

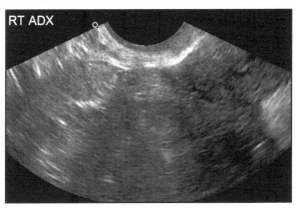

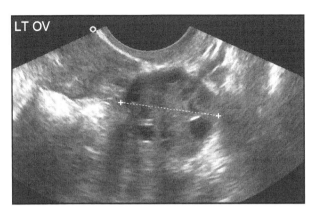

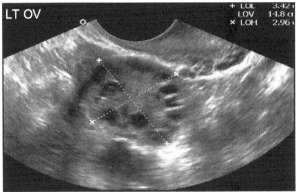

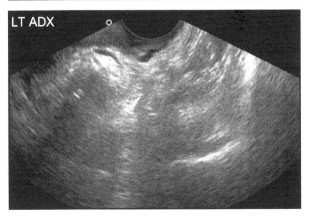

TRANSABDOMINAL

Performed with a **FULL** bladder.

CVX/CDS
UT SAG
UT TRV
ENDO
RT OV TRV
RT OV SAG
LT OV TRV
LT OV SAG

1. Begin in sagital. Note any free-fluid. Evaluate the cervix if it is clearly seen.

2. Measure the uterus in three dimensions. If fibroids are visible, measure the three largest ones and note their locations.

3. Evaluate the endometrium. Measure the anterior to posterior thickness (echogenic stripe to echogenic stripe) and use color Doppler to evaluate its vascularity. Note any visible masses or an IUD if applicable.

4. Measure both ovaries in three dimensions. Measure cysts larger than 2 cm and use color Doppler to evaluate their vascularity.

5. Evaluate the adnexas. Measure any masses and note fluid collections.

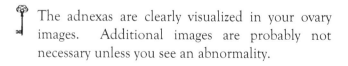 The adnexas are clearly visualized in your ovary images. Additional images are probably not necessary unless you see an abnormality.

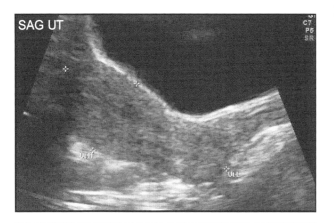

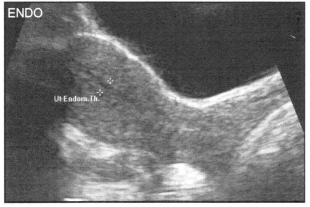

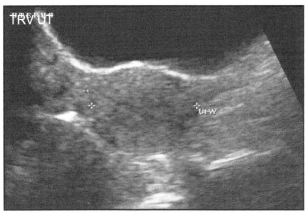

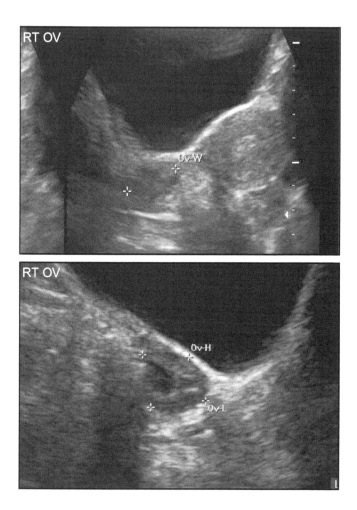

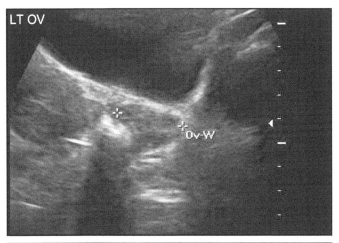

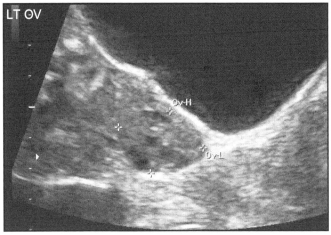

Variants of Uterine Position

Anteverted:

The cervix is parallel with the uterus.

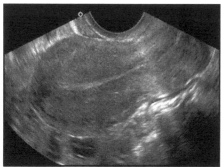 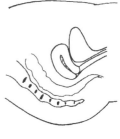

Anteflexed:

The cervix is bent at a 90° angle with the uterus.

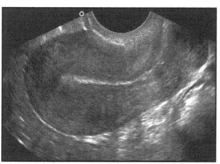 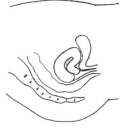

RETROVERTED:

The cervix and uterus are parallel
with the vaginal canal.

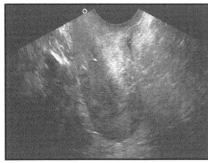 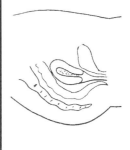

RETROFLEXED:

The uterus is bent posteriorly at the cervix.

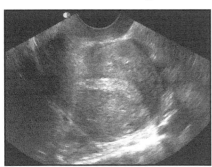 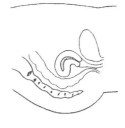

CONGENITAL UTERINE ANOMALIES

Just like human beings, the uterus comes in all shapes and sizes. Some uteruses will be textbook shaped, while others may be a mix of two, making it difficult to determine which category it falls into.

In general, a 3-D image will be the most helpful. If you suspect an abnormality, first determine if the OUTER fundal contour is convex (arched outward) or concave (indented inward). Next you will evaluate the INNER cavity. See the diagram below for more help:

UTERUS	FUNDAL CONTOUR	INNER CONTOUR AND CAVITY
Normal	convex	straight across or convex
Arcuate	convex or mildly concave	indented <1.5 cm
Bicornuate	concave	indented partially or completely to the cervix
Septate	convex	septated completely to the cervix
Subseptate	convex	septated > 1.5 cm

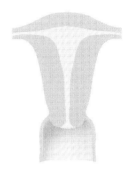

NORMAL UTERUS:

- The fundal contour is convex.
- The inner contour is convex or straight.
- Only one endometrial stripe is observed.

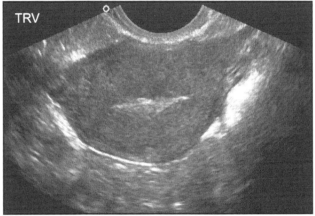

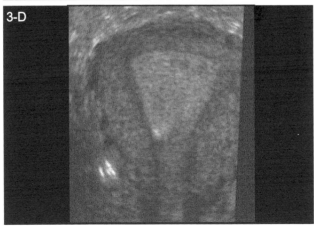

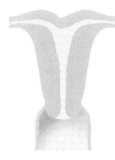

Arcuate Uterus:

- Considered a normal variant.
- The outside fundal contour may be normal or slightly indented.
- The inner contour is indented <1.5 cm into the endometrium.

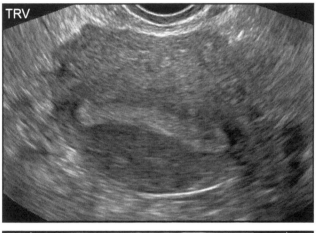

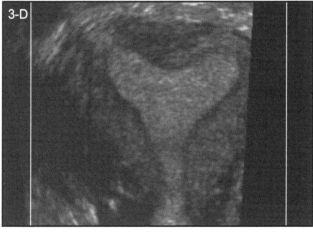

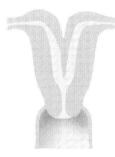

BICORNUATE UTERUS:

- The outer contour is indented >1.5 cm.
- Cervix and vagina are usually single but may be septate or duplicate.
- A didelphys uterus has double uterus, cervix and vagina.

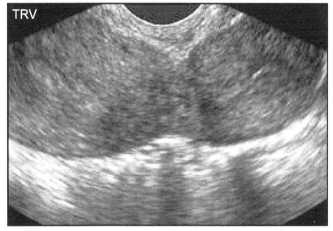

TRV

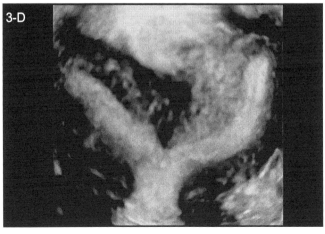

3-D

SEPTATE/SUBSEPTATE UTERUS:

- Outer contour of the fundus appears normal, but the inner cavity is divided by a septum.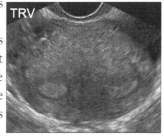
- If the septation extends more than 1.5 cm but less than the entire length of the endometrium, it is considered subseptate.

SEPTATE:

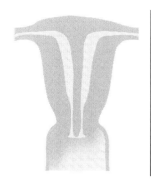 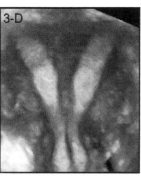

SUBSEPTATE:

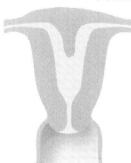 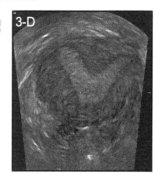

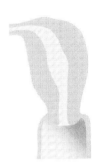

UNICORNUATE UTERUS:

- Singular uterine horn.
- Kidney anomalies are also common.

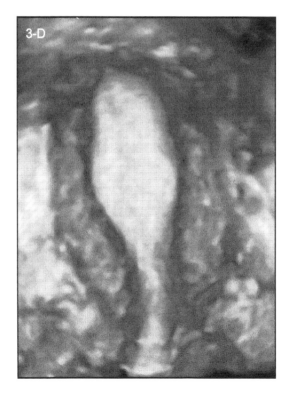

Arcuate Uterus:

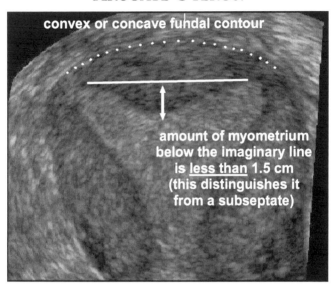

convex or concave fundal contour

amount of myometrium below the imaginary line is _less than_ 1.5 cm (this distinguishes it from a subseptate)

Bicornuate Uterus:

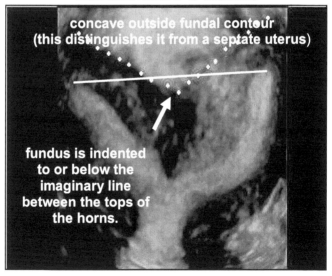

concave outside fundal contour (this distinguishes it from a septate uterus)

fundus is indented to or below the imaginary line between the tops of the horns.

SEPTATE UTERUS:

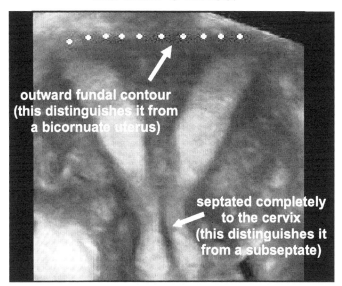

outward fundal contour (this distinguishes it from a bicornuate uterus)

septated completely to the cervix (this distinguishes it from a subseptate)

SUBSEPTATE UTERUS:

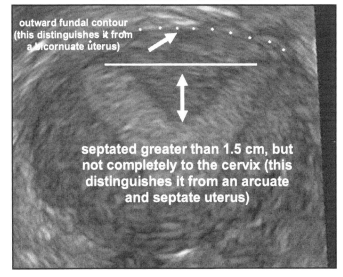

outward fundal contour (this distinguishes it from a bicornuate uterus)

septated greater than 1.5 cm, but not completely to the cervix (this distinguishes it from an arcuate and septate uterus)

PHASES OF THE ENDOMETRIUM

(Measure echogenic stripe to echogenic stripe)

Menstrual

Days: 1-5
Thickness: 2-4 mm

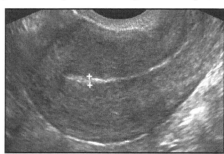

Proliferative

Days: 6-14
Thickness: 5-11 mm

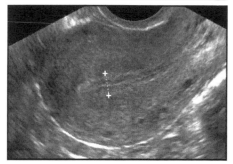

Secretory

Days: 15-28
Thickness: 7-16 mm

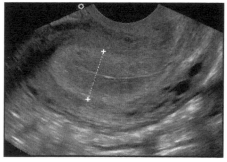

Post Menopausal

< 5 mm or 5-8 mm on hormone therapy
< 6 mm on Tamoxifen

GYNECOLOGICAL FINDINGS

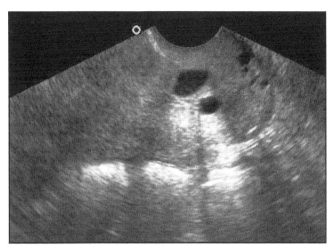

Nabothian cyst: may appear anechoic or hypoechoic, singular or numerous.

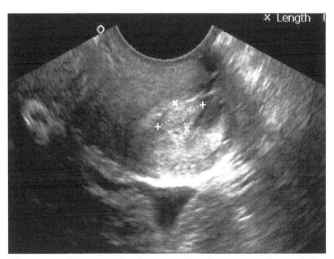

Polyp: this cervical mass had a vascular stalk when observed using color Doppler: *"Cervical mass with vascularity noted."*

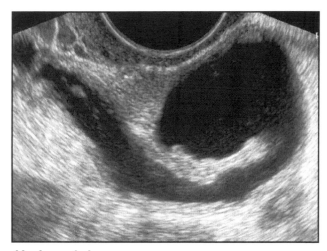

Hydrosalpinx

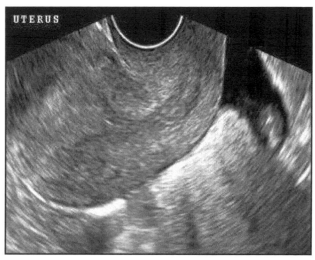

Posterior cul-de-sac fluid

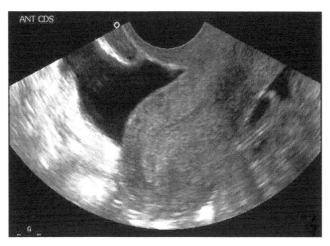

Anterior cul-de-sac fluid: be sure to scan TA as well to assess the amount of fluid in the abdomen. See the image below on the same patient:

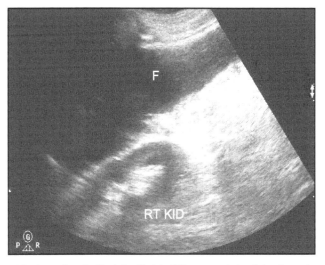

Abdominal fluid: fluid (F) noted in Morison's pouch.

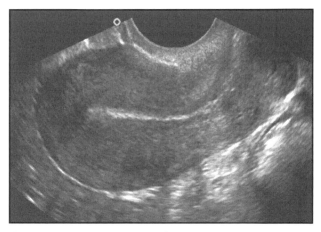

Normal uterus: uniform in shape and thickness anterior and posterior to the endometrium. The texture is homogeneous, medium gray: *"Uterus appears homogeneous with no focal masses."*

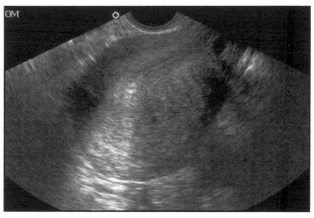

Adenomyosis: posterior fullness, scattered cystic areas, no masses can be clearly seen, endometrium is not well defined: *"Scattered subcentimeter cystic areas and a fullness is noted in the posterior of the uterus."*

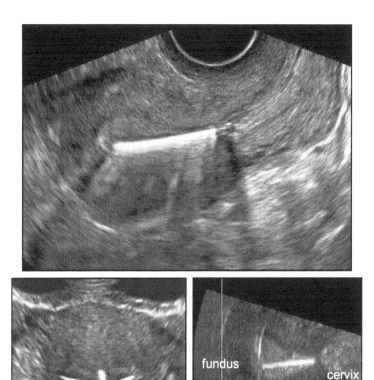

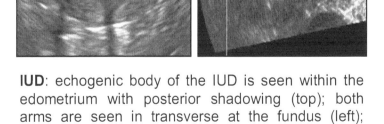

IUD: echogenic body of the IUD is seen within the edometrium with posterior shadowing (top); both arms are seen in transverse at the fundus (left); entire IUD seen in 3D view (right).

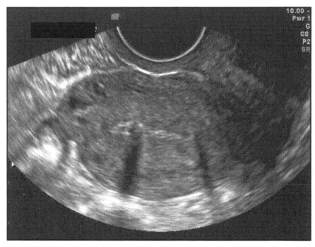

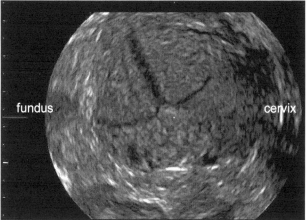

Abnormal IUD: IUD is not positioned in the endometrium.

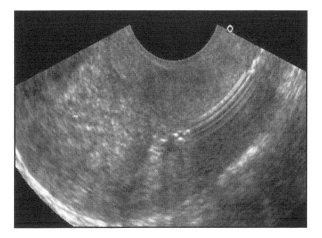

Abnormal IUD: echogenic body is seen in the cervical canal of this uterus. *"IUD is not seen within the endometrium; body appears to be located in the cervical canal."*

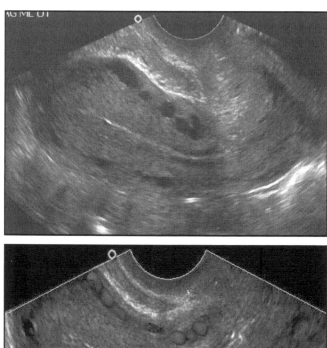

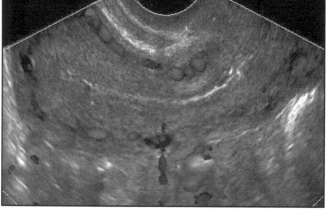

Prominent arcuate arteries: uterus appears to have cystic areas around its rim. Use your color Doppler to determine whether it is prominent arcuate arteries or true cystic areas, which will have no colorflow: *"Hypervascularity is noted around the periphery of the uterus."*

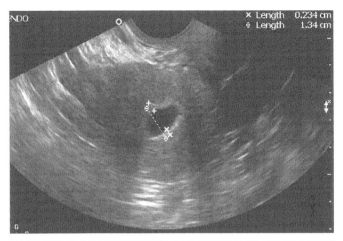

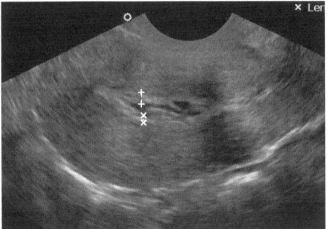

Fluid-filled endometrium: two examples of the correct way to measure the endometrium when fluid is seen within. Add the measurements together for a total endometrial thickness. Note in your report that fluid was seen: *"Moderate amount of fluid is noted within the endometrium."*

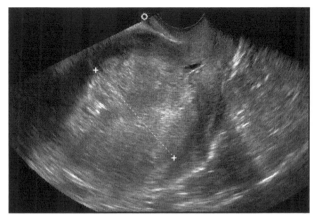

Endometrial hyperplasia, 59.7 mm: post-menopausal patient, atypical cells on biopsy; hysterectomy was scheduled.

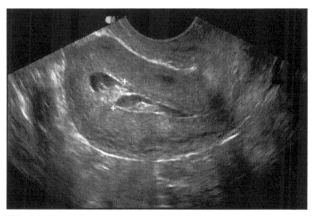

Fluid and debris filled endometrium: measure the total thickness; use color Doppler to evaluate vascularity; clotted blood is non-vascular; retained products of conception are vascular: *"Fluid and debris noted within the endometrial cavity. Contents appears to be non-vascular."*

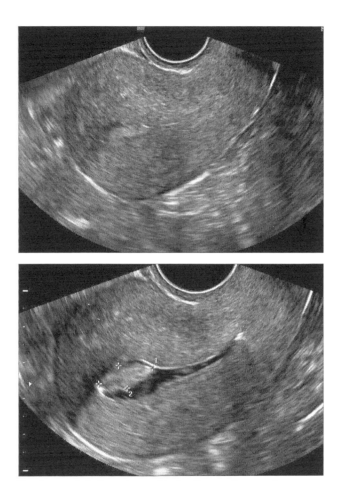

Endometrial polyp: Note the echogenic mass within the endometrium. The mass is easily and more accurately measured during the sonohysterogram procedure seen in the bottom image.

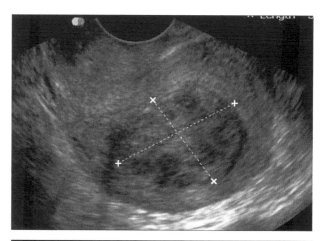

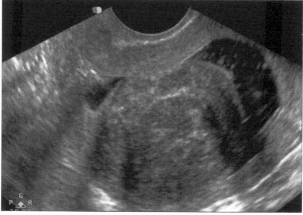

Submucosal fibroid: Large fibroid seen within the endometrium; sonohysterogram helps define the borders.

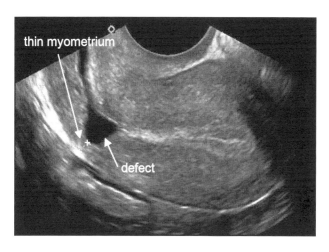

C-section scar dehiscence: the scar has partially separated, also seen in transverse below; myometrium at the defect is thin; patients will need to be closely monitored during future pregnancies.

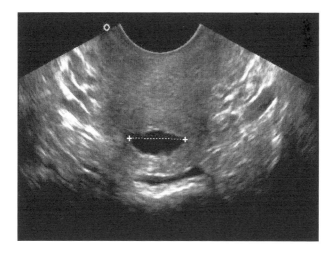

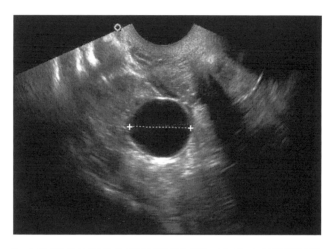

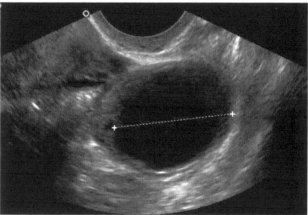

Simple cyst: top image-cyst is anechoic with clearly defined borders; bottom image-cyst is anechoic with hazy borders: "*Simple ovarian cyst noted,*" or "*Mostly clear ovarian cyst noted.*"

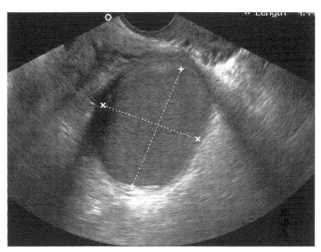

Endometrioma: smooth border and an even gray texture: *"Hypoechoic cyst noted with a homogeneous texture."*

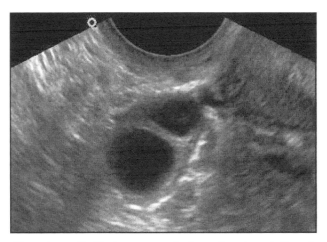

Ovarian follicle: anechoic, clearly defined borders; usually measures less than 2 cm but may become larger.

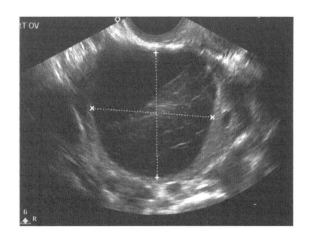

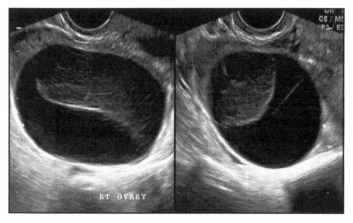

Hemorrhagic cyst with clot: will have the appearance of spider webs.

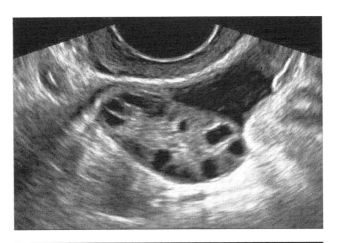

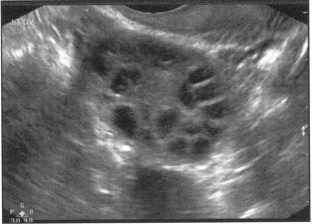

PCOS: ovary appears to have tiny cysts around the perimeter with a "string of pearls" appearance: *"Multiple subcentimeter follicles noted around the perimeter of the ovary with the appearance of PCOS."*

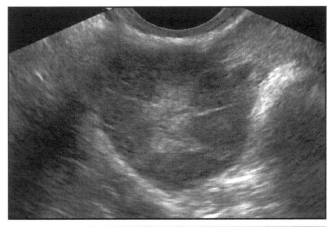

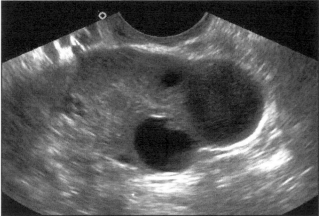

Hyperstimulated ovary: seen with infertility patients; ovaries will appear large and multicystic: *"Bilateral ovarian cysts of varying sizes with the appearance of hyperstimulated ovaries."*

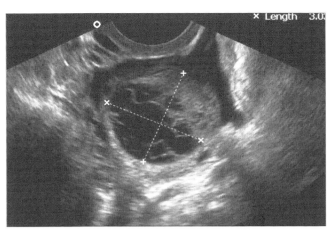

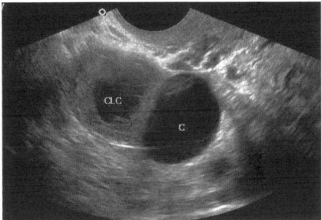

Corpus luteal cyst: appearance will vary depending on how long the cyst has been there, but is usually seen as an anechoic cyst with a thick hypoechoic rim; clot may be seen within; may have a "ring of fire" appearance when viewed using color Doppler, but be careful not to confuse this with an ectopic: *"Mostly clear cyst noted with a hypoechoic rim; has the appearance of a corpus luteal cyst."*

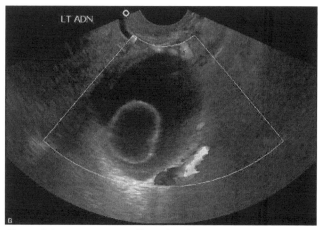

Daughter cyst: smaller simple cyst is seen within a larger cyst; usually benign but may be a sign of malignancy: *"Mostly clear ovarian cyst with daughter cyst; no bloodflow seen within the cyst."*

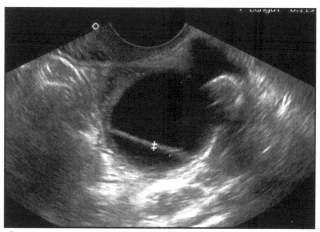

Septated cyst: thin septation noted within a simple cyst; usually benign: *"Simple cyst noted with a thin septation; no bloodflow seen within the cyst."*

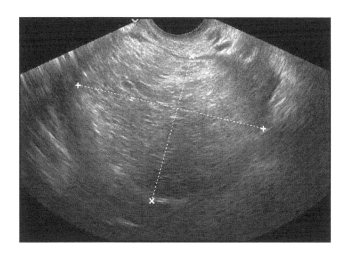

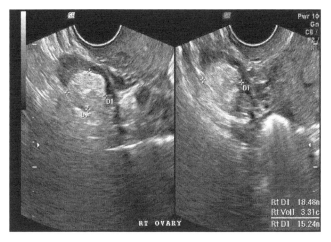

Dermoid: echogenic material is seen within; usually non-vascular: *"Adnexal mass containing echogenic material noted; has the appearance of an ovarian dermoid."*

More examples of dermoid tumors:

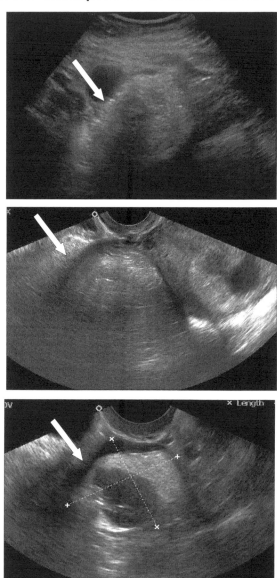

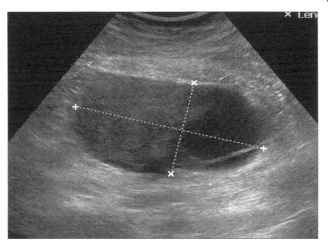

Complex cyst: ovarian cyst seen transabdominally = 10.5 cm in length; family history of breast and renal cancer; CA125 was 234: *"Complex ovarian mass with cystic and solid components."*

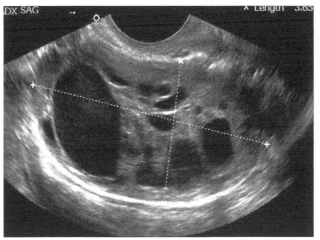

Complex cyst: ovarian cyst = 6.7 cm
"Complex ovarian mass noted with multiple cystic areas."

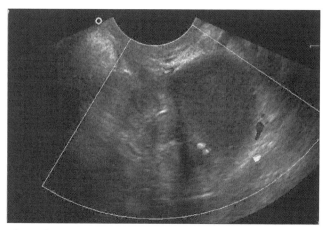

Ovarian tumor: 48 year old with family history of ovarian cancer; CA125 = 296; patient was referred to an oncologist.

<u>Fibroids</u>

Submucosal

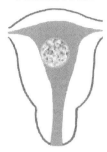
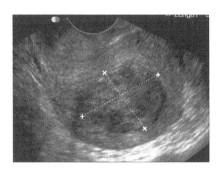

Intramural

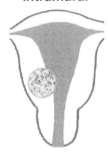
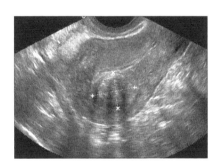

Pedunculated

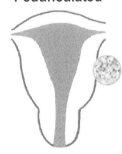
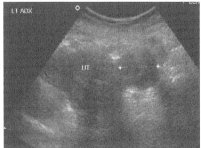

NOTES:

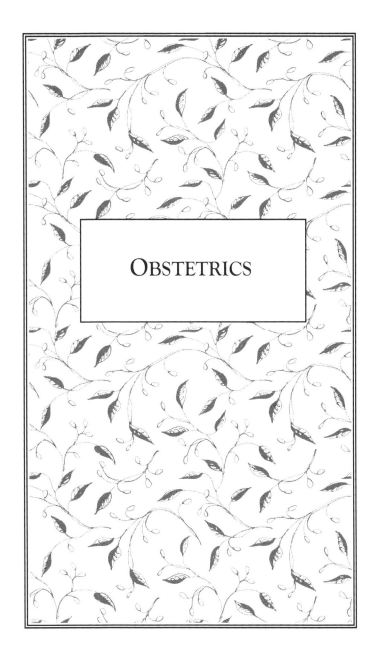

OBSTETRICS

FIRST TRIMESTER

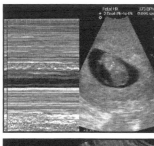
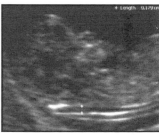
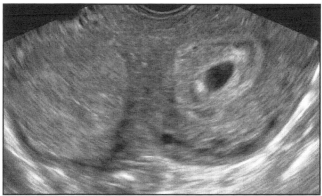

KEY POINTS FOR THE 1ST TRIMESTER:

In the first trimester, the CRL is used to accurately date the pregnancy. Once a date is set, it should not be changed due to subsequent fetal measurements. You will only measure the GS if no fetal pole is seen.

Don't forget to evaluate the perimeter of the gestational sac and measure any subchorionic hemorrhage seen.

If the patient had a positive pregnancy test but you do not see a pregnancy in the uterus (IUP), ectopic should be considered, especially if the beta hCG is >2000 IU. In most cases, an ectopic will be on the same side as the corpus luteal cyst. *"No IUP is seen on today's sonogram. Suboptimal visualization of the adnexas due to overlying bowel and gas. Cannot rule out ectopic at this time."*

If a gestational sac appears to have implanted farther to one side, this may be an interstitial pregnancy. Measure the amount of myometrium between the gestational sac and the outside of the uterus; <5 mm is considered abnormal.

You should see heart motion when the fetus is at least 5 mm (remember: FIVE ALIVE). Always use M-mode in the first trimester to measure the heart rate. Normal rate in the first trimester is between 110-190 bpm.

It is common to see the bowel herniated into the umbilical cord in the first trimester. It will return to its normal location in the abdomen between 12-14 weeks. If bowel is seen outside the abdomen after 15 weeks, gastroschesis or omphalocele should be considered.

1ST TRIMESTER MEASUREMENTS:

- **Gestational sac:**
  visualized at about 5 weeks
  (between 800 - 2000 IU hCG)

- **Yolk sac:**
  visualized at about 5.5 weeks
  (around 2000 IU hCG)
  GS MSD = 8 mm
  YS should measure < 6 mm

- **Embryo:**
  visualized between 5.5 - 6.0 weeks
  GS MSD = 16 mm

- **Cardiac activity:**
  visualized when CRL = 5 mm
  (between 5.5 - 6.0 weeks)

GS cm	Wks/Days	CRL cm
0.2	4w3	
0.3	4w4	
0.4	4w5	
0.5	4w6	
0.6	5w0	
0.7	5w1	
0.8	5w2	
0.9	5w3	
1.0	5w5	0.20
1.1	5w6	0.30
1.2	6w0	0.35
1.3	6w1	0.40
1.4	6w2	0.50
1.5	6w3	0.60
1.6	6w4	0.70
1.7	6w5	0.80
1.8	6w6	0.90
1.9	7w0	0.95
2.0	7w1	1.00
2.1	7w2	1.10
2.2	7w3	1.20
2.3	7w4	1.30
2.4	7w5	1.40
2.5	7w6	1.50
2.6	8w0	1.60

1ST TRIMESTER PROTOCOL

- CVX/CDS–cervix/cul-de-sac
- GS–gestational sac
- YS–yolk sac
- CRL–crown rump length
- HR–heart rate
- RT OV–right ovary
- RT ADX–right adnexa
- LT OV–left ovary
- LT ADX–left adnexa
- CLC–corpus luteal cyst

THE FIRST TRIMESTER SCAN

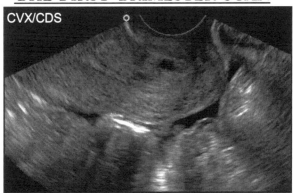

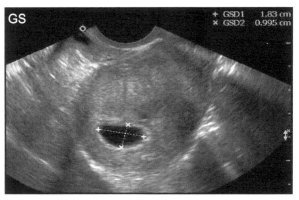

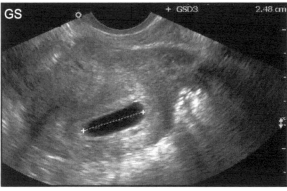

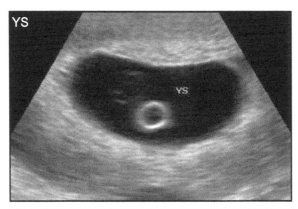

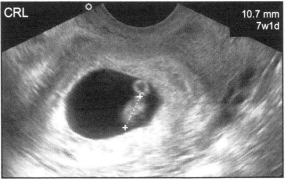

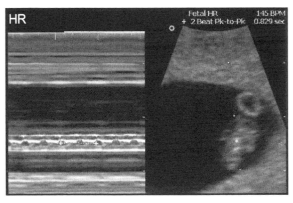

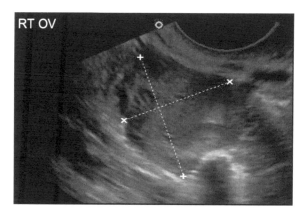

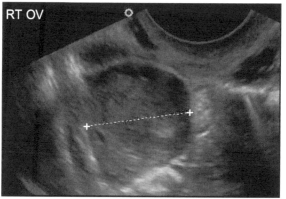

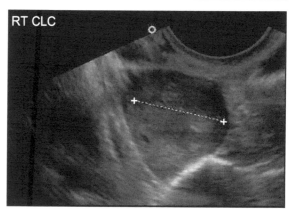

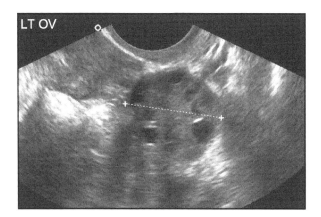

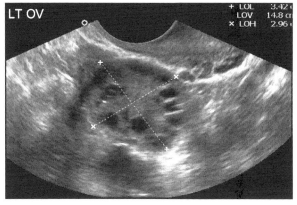

FIRST TRIMESTER SCREENING:

Several tests are available to screen for anomalies in the first trimester. The most common test is the Integrated Screen, which includes the nuchal translucency measurement with blood draw between 11-14 weeks, followed by another blood draw at 16 weeks. The combined result will show the patient's risk of having a fetus with trisomy 21, trisomy 18 and ONTD. The nuchal translucency is measured by a sonographer who is certified to perform this exam. For more information and to become certified, visit www.fetalmedicineusa.com or www.ntqr.org.

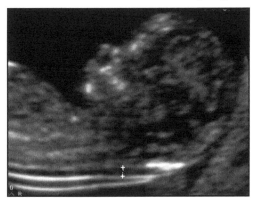

Another test is now available for patients over 35 years of age, called a serum cell free DNA test. It is currently marketed under the names Materni21, Harmony and Panorama. The fetal DNA can now be detected in the maternal blood, which can then be tested for trisomy 13, 18 and 21, however, a blood draw at 16 weeks is still required to check the level of MSAFP. The cell free DNA tests may soon replace the Integrated Screen altogether.

2ND & 3RD
TRIMESTERS

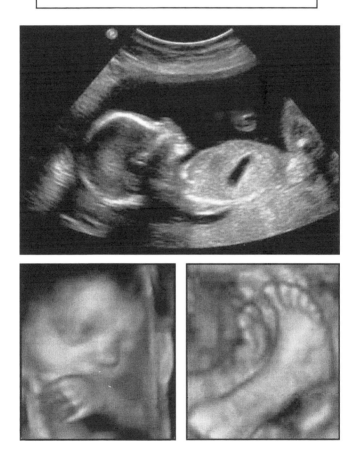

KEY POINTS FOR THE 2ND & 3RD TRIMESTERS:

When performing a 2nd/3rd trimester scan, get in the habit of determining fetal position and normal situs (stomach and heart on left) before anything else.

I recommend always starting with a limited exam, which includes the presentation, placenta, heart rate and AFI. These four images should be included in every 2nd and 3rd trimester scan you perform, even a simple cervical length check.

Always take an image sagitaly at the cervix to show which fetal part is presenting and label it accordingly. It is incorrect to take an image of the fetal head in the fundus and label the image "BREECH". This is the correct label, however you are trying to show the physician which fetal part is presenting at the cervix, not where the head is positioned.

Yawning, fidgeting, nausea and lightheadedness are all signs that your patient's IVC is being compressed. Roll her onto her left side and the symptoms will almost instantly go away.

If your ob patient is presenting with pain, you will want to perform a limited exam, plus a transvaginal cervical length. The patient may not know what a contraction feels like and contractions can cause the cervix to shorten prematurely.

During the second and third trimester, the heart rate should measure between 120-180 bpm. The baby's heart rate will vary depending on its activity level and the amount of caffeine or sugar in the mother's diet.

When measuring the BPD, you should have the third ventricle and thalami in your image, and the calvaria (bones of the skull) will look smooth and symmetric. You should not see the orbits or the cerebellum. The first caliper will be placed on the **outside** of the skull and the second caliper will be placed on the **inside** of the skull. The same image will be used for the HC and your elipse WILL NOT include the fetal skin.

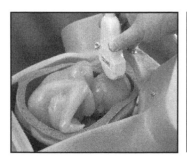 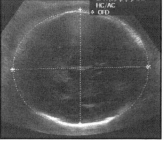

The perfect image of the fetal head becomes more difficult in the late third trimester when it is deep in the maternal pelvis. Try laying the scanning table all the way back and have the patient place her fists under her pelvis. This will elevate the pelvis and help gravity pull the baby toward the fundus.

An easy way to get the correct angle for your BPD/ HC is to get a sagital view of the cervical spine then turn your transducer 90 degrees and slide up through the head.

If you are scanning a fetus with an abnormality, such as hydrocephaly, and cannot see the landmarks, move your transducer superior and inferior until you see the largest circumference and take your measurements there.

Always get a picture of the CSP (cavum septum palucidum). It will appear in the forebrain as an echogenic equal sign, or box. If it is not seen, then agenesis of the corpus callosum must be considered.

The cerebellum will have a peanut or dumbbell shape. If the cerebellum is shaped like a banana (Arnold-Chiari malformation) instead of a peanut, pay careful attention to the spine! Keep in mind that the cerebellar vermis (the part in between the two bulbous areas) will not appear until around 16-17 weeks. Do not confuse this with a Dandy-Walker malformation, where the vermis is partially or totally absent.

When measuring the lateral ventricle, be sure you are measuring the anechoic space of the ventricle and not the echogenic choroid plexus.

The nose/lip image is somewhat difficult to master. Here are a few tips to try: at the level of the 4 chamber heart view, angle your probe towards the fetal head and the nose/lip should appear. Another technique is obtaining the posterior fossa view of the head, then turn your probe 90 degrees and sweep up the face; the nose/lip should appear.

The AC is measured at the level of the stomach and junction of the right and left portal veins. Ribs will be seen symmetric bilaterally. The kidneys should not be visible. Your elipse WILL include the fetal skin.

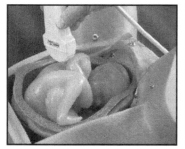
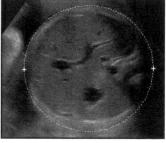

Keep in mind that the accuracy of the fetal weight estimate decreases as the pregnancy progresses into the third trimester and a ± 15% variation may occur.

If the HC and femur measure normal but the AC is measuring small, this may indicate placental insufficiency; if all the measurements are small, this may indicate a chromosomal abnormality.

If you suspect echogenic bowel, decrease gain until you only see bone, then determine if the bowel is truly echogenic.

An easy way to tell if the orbits are normally spaced is to imagine adding a third orbit between the two existing orbits; if it fits, then you can rule out hypotelorism.

Try to get a longitudinal shot of the fetal abdomen showing the heart, diaphragm, stomach and bladder. This shows these organs are in their correct locations and rules out a diaphragmatic hernia.

Landmarks for transverse spine images: cervical spine is superior to the heart near the clavical bones; thoracic spine is at the level of the heart; lumbar spine is at the level of the kidneys; sacrum is near the bladder at the iliac bones.

Clear spine images are important for ruling out spina bifida and scoliosis. If the posterior fossa of the brain appears normal, the fetus most likely does not have spina bifida. If possible, try to get the fetus away from the uterine wall so you can see a smooth skin line and an evenly aligned spinal column to rule out scoliosis.

Always be sure you see the umbilical arteries connect at the abdominal wall interface. It is easy to mistake an iliac vessel for an umbilical artery and miss diagnosing a two vessel cord. *Remember: 3 vessel cord = 2 arteries, 1 vein; 2 vessel cord = 1 artery, 1 vein.

☙ Be sure the arms have both a radius and ulna, as well as both hands. The ulna is longer than the radius and extends to the elbow.

☙ A correct femur measurement is taken when the femur is parallel or slightly oblique to the ultrasound beam.

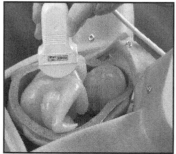 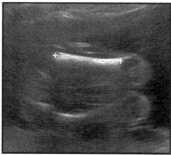

☙ A femur measuring 7 or more days less than the gestational age is a soft marker for Down syndrome.

☙ A correct image of the lower leg will include the fibula and tibia. The tibia is longer than the fibula and will extend to the knee. The foot will appear round because it is pointing at you. If you see both lower leg bones and the side of the foot in the same plane, careful evaluation for club foot is necessary.

☙ Fluid in the renal pelvis is called pyelectasis. When the fluid is also seen in the renal calyces, it is called hydronephrosis.

☙ "Keyhole" appearance of the bladder is caused by posterior urethral valves (PUV), seen only in males.

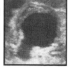

If you suspect a horseshoe kidney, get a coronal view and turn on your color Doppler; the aorta and IVC will appear to be interrupted due to the connection of the two kidneys at either the superior or inferior poles.

If you see hydronephrosis in only half the kidney (i.e. the upper pole), there may be a duplicated collecting system.

Large, echogenic kidneys with no visible bladder may be signs of ARPKD (autosomal recessive polycystic kidney disease). If one of the kidneys has anechoic cysts of varying sizes, MCDK (multicystic dysplastic kidney) must be considered.

Most common cause of urinary tract dilatation is UPJ (ureter pelvic junction) obstruction, which causes fluid to back up into the kidney.

Using color Doppler on the renal arteries will help prove there are two kidneys.

If a second or third trimester patient presents with bleeding, be sure to check the placenta carefully for abruption, which may appear as a fluid filled collection or heterogeneous mass beneath the placenta or at the margins.

Try to avoid guessing the gender before 16 weeks. If you do take a guess, remind the patient that it is ONLY a guess.

When you are performing a BPP, keep in mind the amount of time it takes the fetus to do the required parameters. A sluggish baby could mean something isn't right. If it takes the full 30 minutes for the baby to breathe or move, mention this to the obstetrician. It's better to play it safe.

If feasible, try to have a second set of eyes review your images if you suspect an abnormality.

You may get a concerned mother when the heart rates of her twins are different. Reassure her they are two different little people and their heart rates will differ.

It is not always possible to obtain the perfect image; know when it is time to move on.

Be sure to document not only what you see, but also what you DON'T see. Reasons may be due to position or body habitus, but you are ultimately responsible for the images you take or fail to take.

2nd & 3rd Trimester Measurements

- **Cervical length:** should measure at least 2.5 cm

- **Lateral ventricle:** < 10mm

- **Cisterna magna:** < 10mm

- **AFI:** <5 cm = oligohydramnios
    >25 cm = polyhydramnios

- **Tachycardia:** >180 bpm

- **Bradycardia:** <100 bpm

- **Low lying placenta:** placenta is <2.0 cm from the internal os.

- **Placentomegaly:** >4.5 cm thickness

- **Renal pelvis:** ≤ 3 mm in the first trimester
    ≤ 4 mm between 14-22 weeks
    ≤ 5 mm between 22-32 weeks
    ≤ 7 mm after 32 weeks

- **Bladder:**   < 3 cm diameter in 2nd trimester
    < 5 cm in the third trimester
    ≥ 6 cm is megacystis

- **IUGR:** EFW <10% and AC is <25%

- **Brachychephaly:** BPD is large for gestational age, ratio is >85.

- **Dolichocephaly:** OFD is large for gestational age, ratio is <70, common in breech and when the head is deep in the lower uterine segment.

FETAL LENGTHS

GA Weeks	Length in inches	Size of a:
8	1.5	raspberry
10	2.4	prune
12	3.5	plum
14	4.7	lemon
16	6.25	avocado
18	7.8	sweet potato
20	9.75	banana
22	11	papaya
24	11.7	cantaloupe
26	12.5	lettuce
28	13.65	eggplant
30	14.8	cucumber
32	15.6	squash
34	16.4	butternut squash
36	17.5	coconut
38	18.7	honeydew
40	19.5	watermelon

.

PROTOCOLS FOR
2ND & 3RD TRIMESTERS

BIOPHYSICAL PROFILE (BPP)

Each parameter is scored a 2 (normal)
or 0 (abnormal) in 30 minutes:

- BREATHING—15 seconds
- MOVEMENT— three gross body movements
- TONE— hand or limb bending and straightening
- AFI— >2 cm in a single vertical pocket

Non-stress test may be included and will show two fetal
heart accelerations of >15 BPM in 20 minutes.

Keep in mind when watching the diaphragm for breathing, you may see it moving due to heart motions; when in doubt, obtain a coronal view of the kidneys; they will appear to slide up and down with true fetal breathing movements due to pressure from the diaphragm.

LIMITED

- FETAL LIE—cephalic, breech or transverse
- PL SAG—placenta sagital
- PL TRV—placenta transverse
- PL CI—placenta cord insert
- HR—heart rate
- AFI—amniotic fluid index

ANATOMY

Limited PLUS:

- SP SAG—spine sagital
- SP TRV—spine transverse
- HC/BPD—head circumference/biparietal diameter
- CB/CM/NF—cerebellum, cisterna magna, nuchal fold
- LV—lateral ventricle
- CP—choroid plexus
- CSP—cavum septum palucidum
- N/L—nose, lips
- ORBITS
- PROFILE
- UPPER EXT—upper extremity (both)
- HAND (both)
- 4CH—four chamber heart
- LVOT—left ventricular outflow tract
- RVOT—right ventricular outflow tract
- AC—abdominal circumference
- KIDNEYS
- CI—cord insert
- 3VC—three vessel cord
- FL—femur length
- LOWER EXT—lower extremity (both)
- FOOT (both)
- HT/ST/BL—heart, stomach, bladder
- GENDER

FETAL ANOMALIES TO RULE OUT DURING THE ANATOMY SCAN:

head circumference	anencephaly, exencephaly, encephalocele, lemon sign (spina bifida), scalp edema, cloverleaf shape
lateral ventricle	ventriculomegaly
cavum septum pelucidum	agenesis of the corpus callosum
Posterior fossa (cerebellum, cisterna magna, nuchal fold)	banana sign (spina bifida), large cisterna magna, Dandy-Walker malformation (includes ventriculomegaly, especially the fourth ventricle, absence of cerebellar vermis, and cyst formation near the lowest part of the skull).
orbits	hypo or hypertelorism, anophthalmia/ cyclopia
nose and upper lip	cleft lip
profile	absent or flat nose, micrognathia, proboscis
spine	cystic hygroma, spina bifida, sacral teratoma, neck masses
4 chamber heart transverse chest	situs abnormality, cardiomegaly, septal defects, arrhythmia, pericardial effusion, deformed ribs, pleural effusion, lung masses
LVOT/RVOT	overriding aorta, transposition of the great arteries

diaphragm	heart and stomach are on opposite sides to rule out herniation
transverse abdomen	stomach on the left side, duodenal atresia, ascites
kidneys	hydronephrosis/pyelectasis, agenesis, hydroureter, duplication, pelvic kidney, multicystic or polycystic kidneys
fetal cord insertion	gastroschisis, omphalocele, limb-body wall complex, cord mass
urinary bladder	umbilical cord vessel number, agenesis, outlet obstruction, exstrophy, posterior uretheral valves (males only)
upper extremities	shortened or absent radius, dwarfism, amputation, edema, fractures, polydactyly (extra digits), syndactyly (webbed digits)
lower extremities	dwarfism, amputation, clubfoot, edema, fractures, polydactyly (extra digits), syndactyly (webbed digits)

THE ANATOMY SCAN

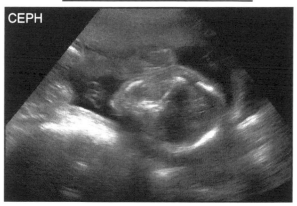

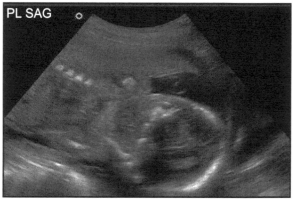

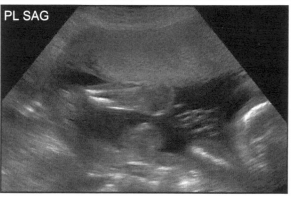

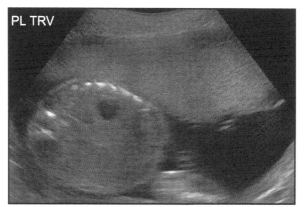

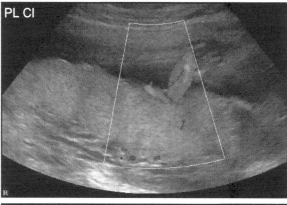

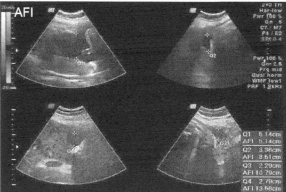

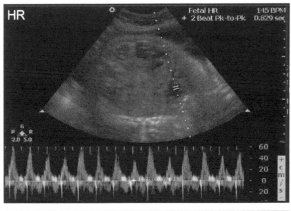

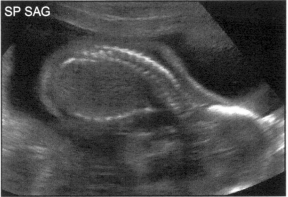

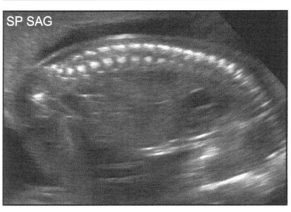

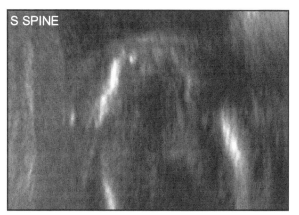

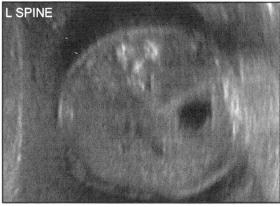

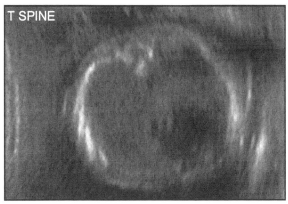

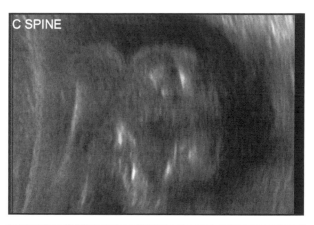

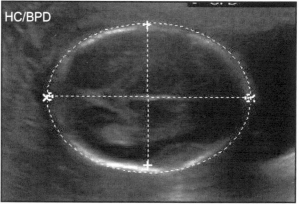

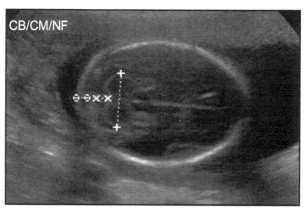

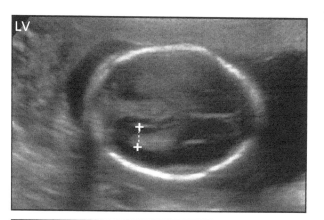

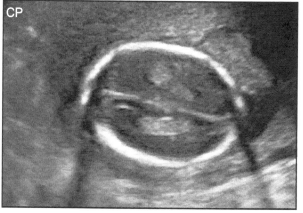

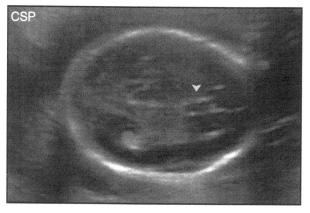

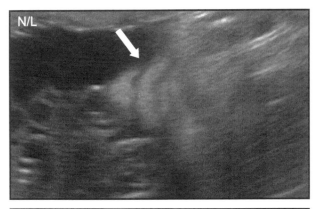

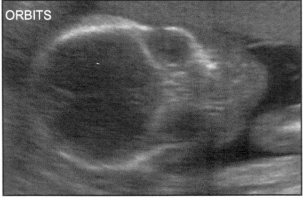

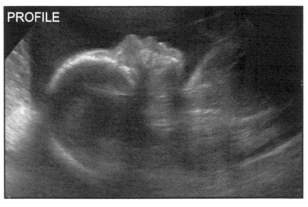

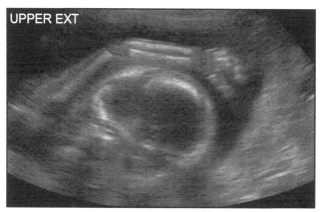

UPPER EXT

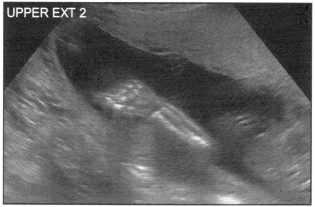

UPPER EXT 2

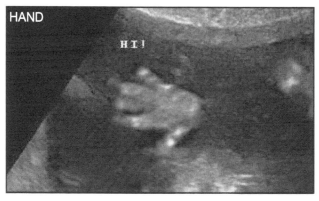

HAND

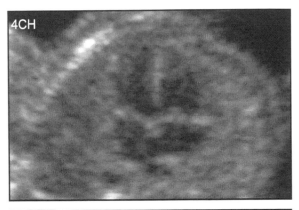

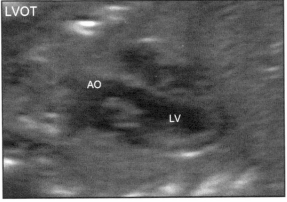

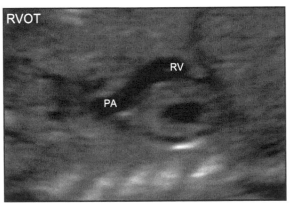

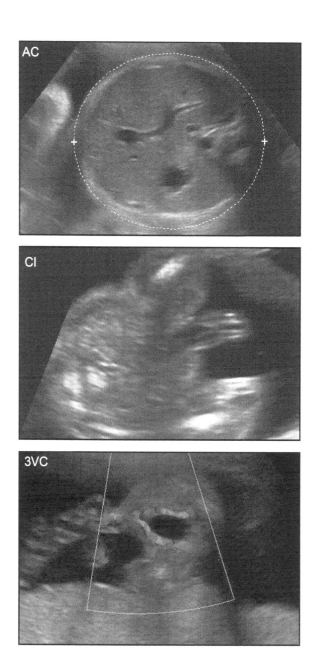

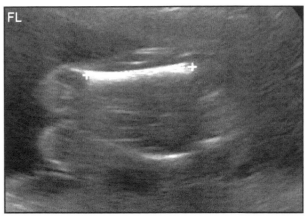

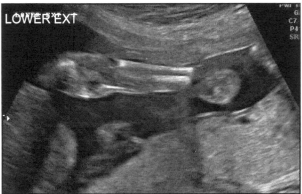

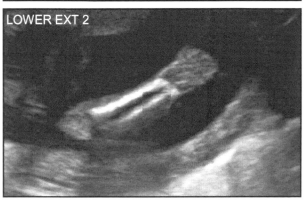

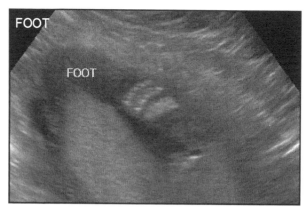

FOOT

FOOT

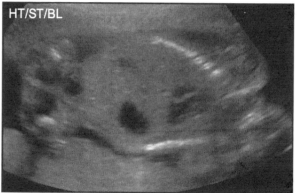

HT/ST/BL

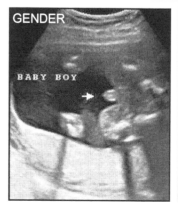

GENDER

BABY BOY

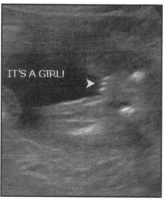

IT'S A GIRL!

THE FETAL ENVIRONMENT

PLACENTA

CERVIX

AMNIOTIC FLUID

PLACENTA

Think of the placenta as a filter for the fetus. It allows oxygen and nutrients to pass through from the mother's blood and removes waste from the fetal environment. When you are evaluating the placenta your goal is to rule out:

- Improper umbilical cord insertion

- Placenta previa, accreta, increta, percreta

- Premature aging (calcification) of the placenta

- Succenturiate placenta (additional piece of placenta)

- Start at the edge closest to the cervix, then take one or two more images of the mid section and one of the far edge, followed by an image in transverse. Use color Doppler to help locate the cord insertion.

- If a bleed is noted against the maternal surface of the placenta it is called a subchorionic hemorrhage or hematoma. If it is seen within the placenta it is called a placental lake, and if you see bubble on the fetal surface of the placenta, it is a subamniotic hemorrhage.

- The placental thickness should measure between 2-4 cm. If it appears thickened, be sure your transducer is perpendicular to the placenta and not at an oblique angle or you might falsely increase placental thickness.

LOCATIONS OF THE PLACENTA

The fetus, placenta and uterus are continuously growing during pregnancy and the placenta will move due to the growth of the uterus. The placenta may be located anterior, posterior, fundal, right or left lateral, or any combination of these.

- An anterior placenta will be seen at the top of the screen.

- A posterior placenta will be seen at the bottom of the screen.

- In sagital, a fundal placenta will be at the left side of the screen.

- A previa placenta will completely cover the internal os.

- A partial previa will only cover a small portion of the internal os.

- A low-lying placenta will measure less than 2.0 cm from the internal os.

- Anterior placentas more often move away from the internal os than do posterior placentas due to the growing uterus.

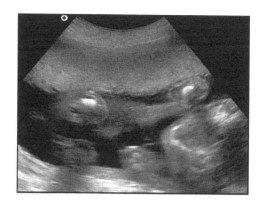

Anterior

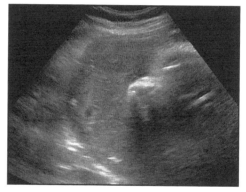

Fundal

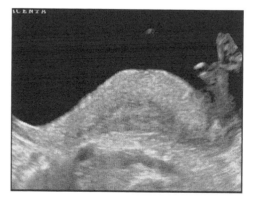

Posterior

GRADING THE PLACENTA

The amount of calcifications you see in the placenta will determine its grade. There are four numbers used to grade placentas: 0, 1, 2 and 3. In general, the older the placenta, the more calcifications present, but this is not always the case. See the images on the next page for more information.

When a placenta is thought to be aging too rapidly (many calcifications), common in high blood pressure, diabetic patients and maternal cigarette smoking, the baby's growth will be monitored to be sure he is getting enough nutrients. In addition, oligohydramnios may be caused by placental insufficiency, so the amniotic fluid level is also checked frequently. Some doctors do not feel it is necessary to grade the placenta. Refer to your site's ultrasound manual for the appropriate protocol.

Doppler assessments are also used to assess placental insufficiency, however, this book will not cover this procedure.

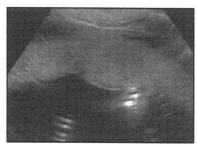

Grade 0: <18 weeks

- Uniform echogenicity
- Smooth chorionic plate
- No indentations

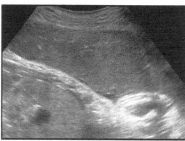

Grade 1: 18-29 weeks

- Few calcifications
- Subtle indentations

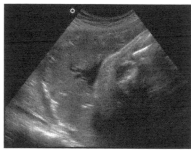

Grade 2: 30-38 weeks

- Mild calcifications in parenchyma
- Larger indentations
- Calcifications along the chorionic plate

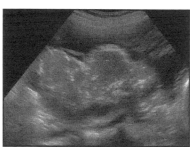

Grade 3: >38 weeks

- Significant clacifications
- Lobules are seen
- Fetal surface is irregular

PLACENTAL CORD INSERT SITES

Normally, the umbilical cord will insert into the center of the placenta. Insertion towards the edge of the placenta is called an **eccentric cord insertion** and usually causes no problems for the fetus; insertion on the chorionic membranes instead of into the placenta is called **velamentous cord insertion**. In this condition, the vessels travel between the amnion and chorion to the placenta and are not protected by Wharton's jelly, which means they can easily rupture. If they travel across the cervix, it is called **vasa previa** and can be life threatening to the mother and fetus.

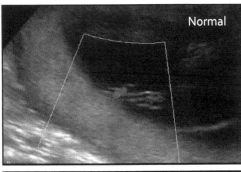

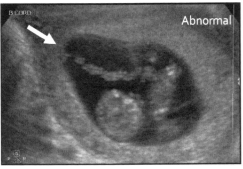

ABNORMAL PLACENTAL ATTACHMENT

In a normal placental attachment, you will see a hypoechoic division between the placenta and the uterus, and the bladder wall appears smooth. If your patient has an anterior low-lying or previa placenta and any risk factors for placenta accreta (previous c-section, placenta previa, fibroids, any conditions causing myometrial tissue damage), you will need to evaluate the placenta/uterine interface at approximately 20 weeks.

If the patient has had one previous c-section, there is about a 10% chance of placenta accreta. If the patient has had more than one c-section, the chance of placenta accreta can be as high as 40%.

Clues to diagnose placenta accreta:

The placenta may have a Swiss cheese look, called vascular lacunae, a loss of hypoechoic myometrium between the placenta and bladder, or a loss of the smooth echogenic bladder wall. With a cervical placenta accreta, you will not see a smooth border between the cervix and placenta; using color Doppler, you may see blood flowing between the placenta and cervix.

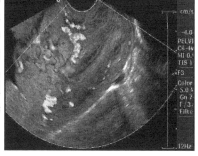

CERVIX

For patients at risk for preterm labor, serial cervical measurements are usually started at 16 weeks and will continue until 28 weeks. The cervical length should measure 2.5 cm or more. Proper and consistent technique is vital.

- Visualize the internal and external os. The internal os is difficult to distinguish from the lower uterine segment in the early second trimester. The internal os will usually be just posterior to the echogenic stripe of the peritoneum between the bladder and uterine wall (see images on next page).

- Decrease your pressure to ensure the anterior and posterior segments are of equal thickness.

- Begin your measurement at the internal os and continue the measurement to the external os.

- Apply fundal pressure to simulate gravity and re-measure.

- Be sure to note any funneling observed at the internal os. Your site may require you to measure the width and depth of the funneling.

- If your patient has a cerclage in place, it will appear as an echogenic foci in the anterior and posterior portions of the cervical body in sagittal. In transverse it will look like an echogenic circle or lasso.

NON-PREGNANT UTERUS

Notice that the endometrium is continuous with the cervical canal and it is difficult to determine where the internal os (IO) is located. In early pregnancy, the lower uterine segment (LUS) is still quite thick and remains clamped down on the internal os. By 16 weeks, it still may be difficult to see the IO, but if you use the line of echogenic peritoneum that divides the uterus and bladder to guide you, your measurement will be more accurate. Simply draw an imaginary line perpendicular to the endometrial stripe from the peritoneum and this is the division between the LUS and IO. More examples are on the next few pages.

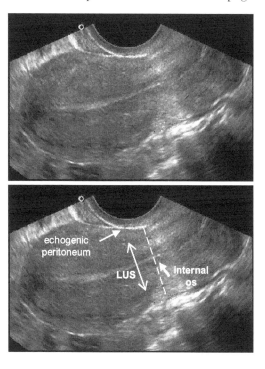

Cervix at 8 weeks gestation

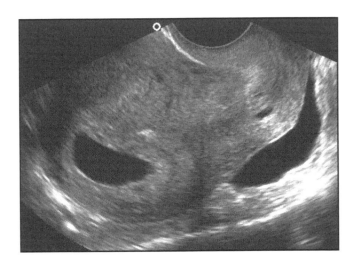

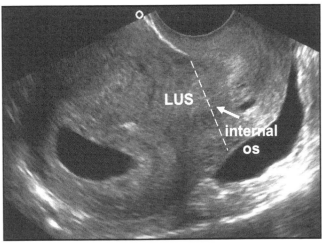

CERVIX AT 16 WEEKS GESTATION

Serial cervical measurements are usually started during week 16. Notice that the LUS remains thick at this stage.

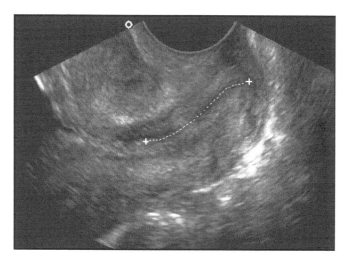

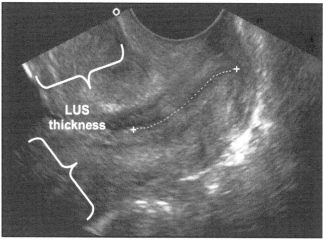

CERVIX AT 20 WEEKS GESTATION
Notice how the lower uterine segment has really thinned out, revealing the internal os.

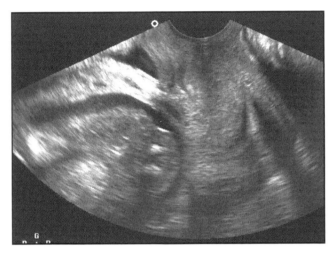

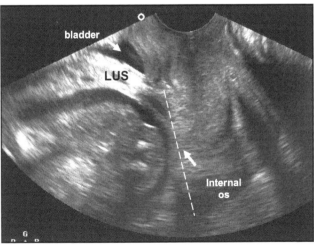

INCOMPETENT CERVIX

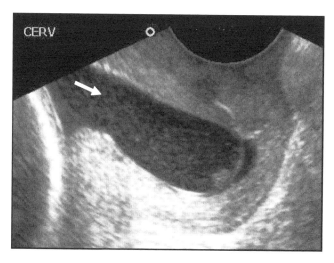

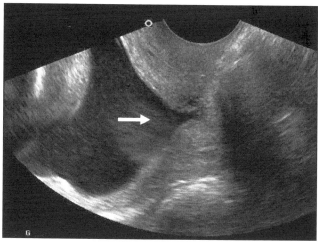

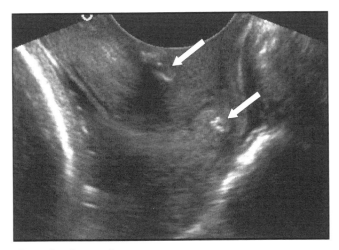

Cervical cerclage

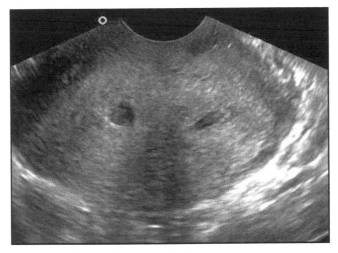

Septated cervix: seen in transverse.

AMNIOTIC FLUID INDEX

- Divide the belly into four quadrants at the navel and measure the deepest vertical pocket in each quadrant.

- Keep your transducer perpendicular to the floor at all times.

- Use color Doppler to ensure you are not measuring through umbilical cord.

- Take the 4 AFI quadrants in the same order every time so you don't forget which ones you have already done.

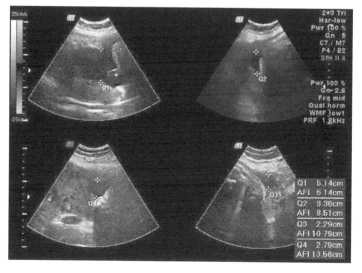

Remember: you cannot do an AFI on twins. Measure the deepest vertical pocket in each sac.

OBSTETRICAL FINDINGS

This is just a small sampling of what you may find during an ob exam. Check the back of this book for more sources.

ECTOPIC PREGNANCY:

If a patient had a positive pregnancy test and you do not see an IUP, think ECTOPIC. An early gestational sac will be fairly round or oval in sagital and transverse and will have an echogenic ring around it called the decidual sign. A "pseudo sac" will just be a collection of fluid, usually more irregular in shape.

Pay careful attention to the side of the pelvis with the corpus luteal cyst. The ectopic will be on this side 85% of the time. If you see a cystic area in the adnexa, use color Doppler to look for fetal heart beats. Corpus luteal cysts and ectopic masses can look very similar. The key is to determine if the mass is on the ovary or in the adnexa. Apply pelvic pressure to see if the mass moves independent of the ovary.

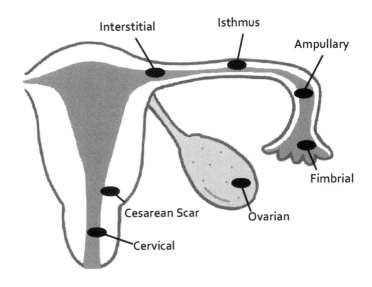

Clues of a possible ectopic pregnancy:

- Positive pregnancy test and no IUP seen
- Fluid in the cul-de-sac
- Pain with pelvic pressure
- An adnexal mass that moves independent of the ovary

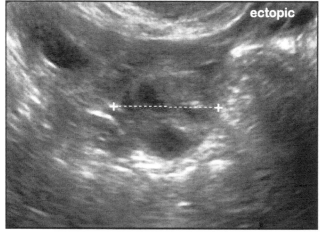

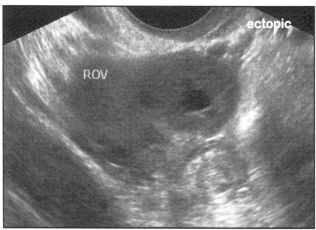

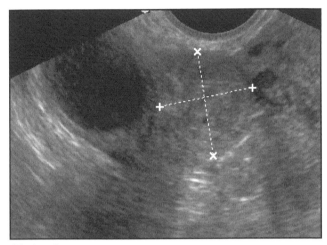

Ectopic pregnancy

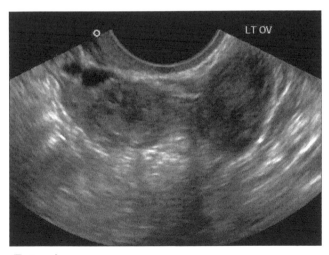

Ectopic pregnancy

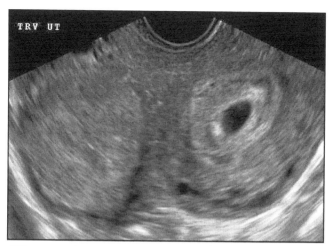

Bicornuate pregnancy: seen in the left horn.

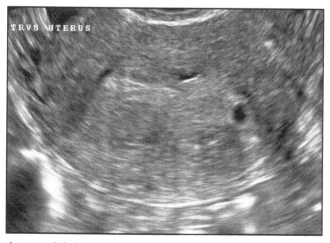

Interstitial pregnancy: gestational sac in the left interstitial area of the uterus.

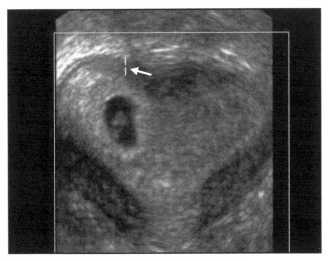

Arcuate uterus with gestational sac: be sure there is at least 5 mm of myometrium at the edge of the sac.

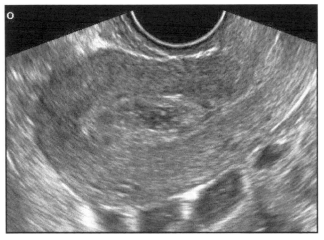

Retained products of conception (RPOC): use color Doppler to assess vascularity; a blood clot will have no vascularity.

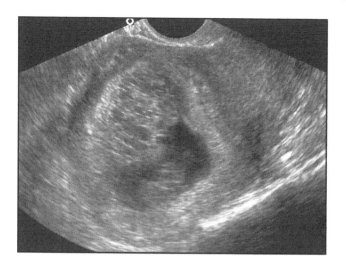

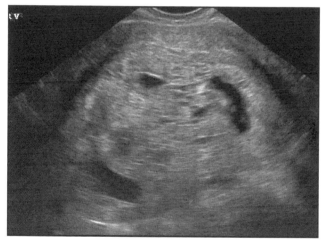

Molar pregnancy: notice the complex endometrium with multiple cystic spots, commonly known as the "cluster of grapes" appearance. Serial blood tests are required to ensure the hCG level returns to negative.

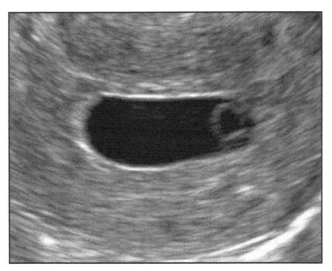

Normal gestational sac

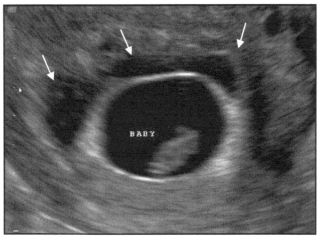

Gestational sac with subchorionic hemorrhage.

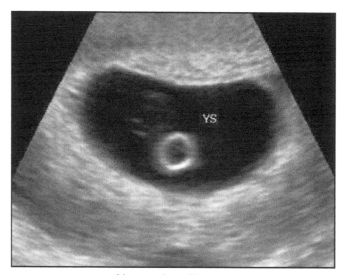

Normal yolk sac

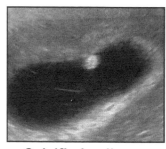

Calcified yolk sac

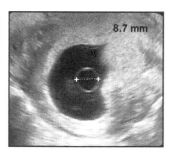

Large yolk sac

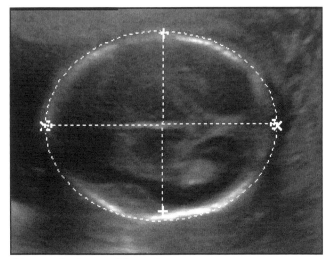

Normal shaped head

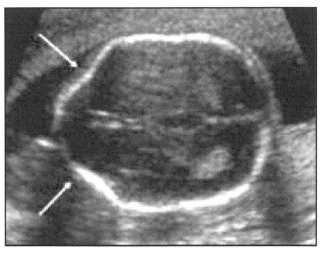

Abnormal lemon-shaped head (evaluate the spine closely for spina bifida).

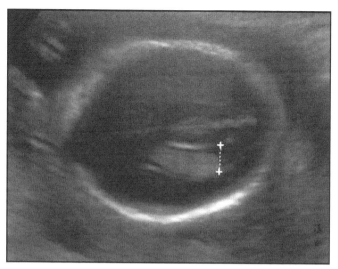

Lateral ventricle: location of measurement is correct in the image above.

Incorrect measurement of the lateral ventricle: the calipers in the images on the right are placed on either side of the choroid plexus.

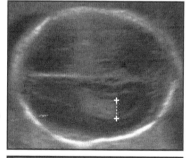

Remember, you are measuring the space in which the choroid plexus resides, not the echogenic choroid plexus itself.

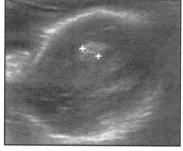

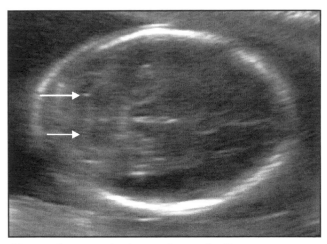

Normal peanut-shaped cerebellum

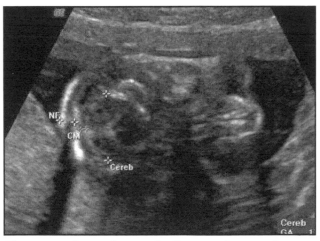

Banana-shaped cerebellum: abnormal; pay close attention to the spine.

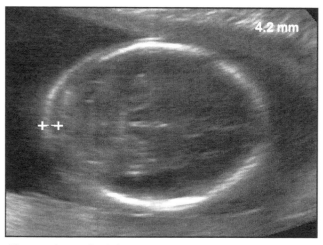

Normal nuchal fold = <6mm thickness

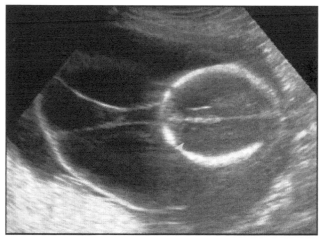

Nuchal fold with cystic hygroma

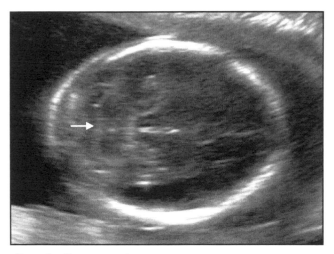

Cerebellar vermis

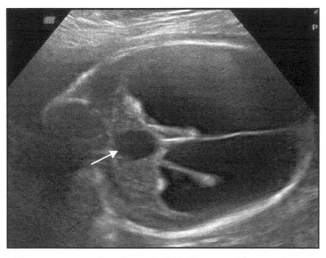

Absent vermis: Dandy Walker malformation

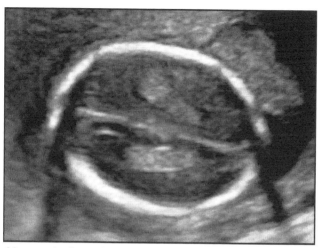

Normal choroid plexus

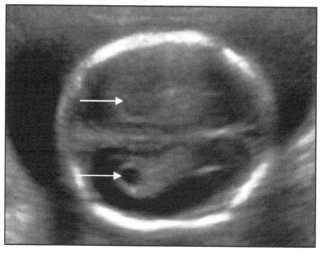

Choroid plexus cysts

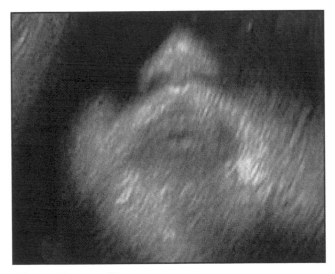

Normal nose/lip

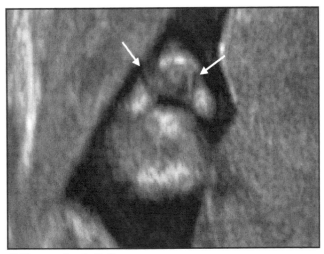

Bilateral cleft lip

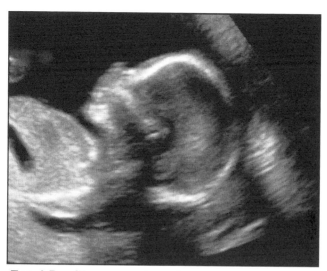

Fetal Profile: correct angle

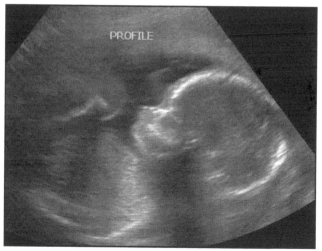

Incorrect view of fetal profile: unable to
evaluate chin for micrognathy.

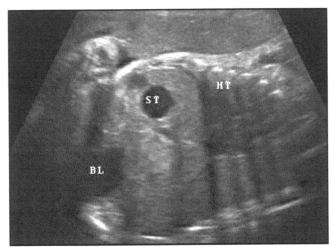

Normal bowel, sagital

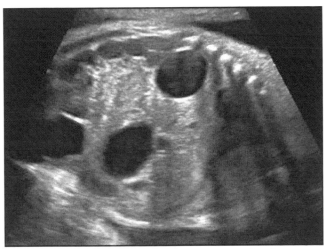

Duodenal atresia (double bubble sign), may also be seen in transverse.

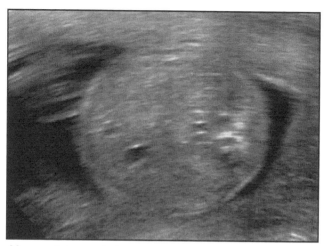

Normal bowel, transverse

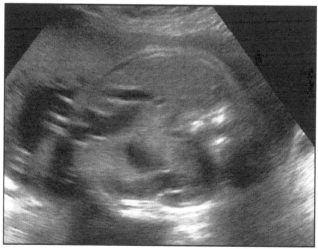

Dilated bowel

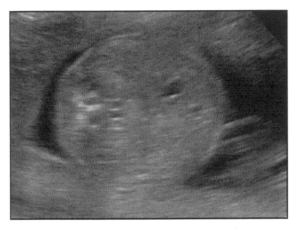

Normal bowel, transverse view

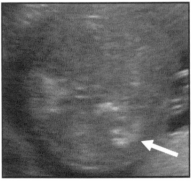

Echogenic bowel, 2nd Trimester

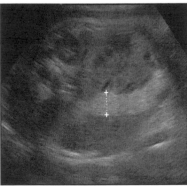

Echogenic bowel, 3rd Trimester

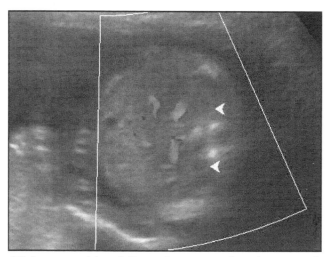

Kidneys: blood-flow is seen in the renal arteries.

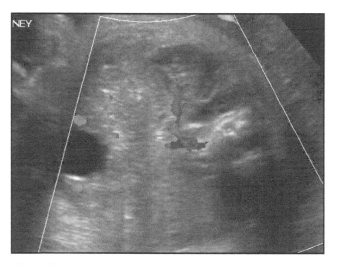

Renal agenesis: blood-flow is seen only in the single renal artery.

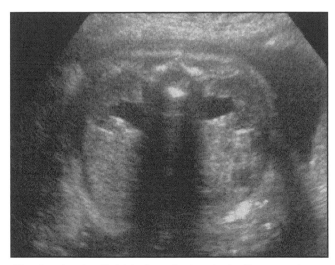

Pyelectasis-fluid is located only in the renal pelvis.

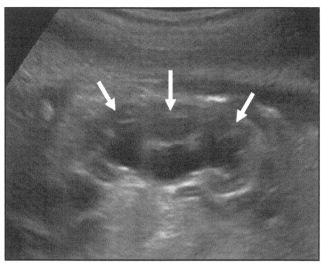

Hydronephrosis-fluid is noted in the renal pelvis as well as the calyces.

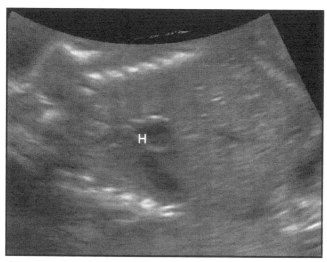

Normal fetal chest; (H=heart)

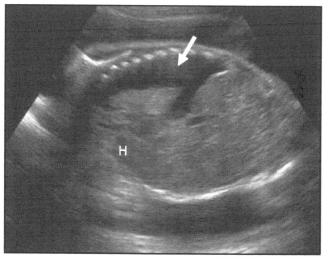

Pleural effusion; (H=heart)

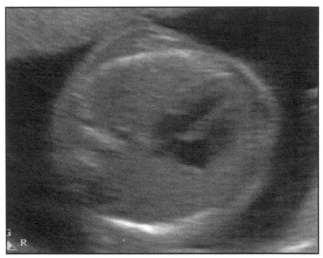

Normal fetal chest in transverse

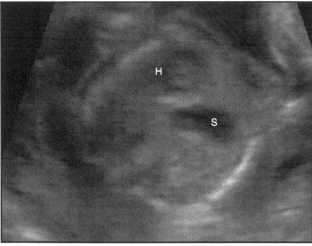

Abnormal fetal chest: heart and stomach are seen in the same transverse view, consistent with diaphragmatic hernia.

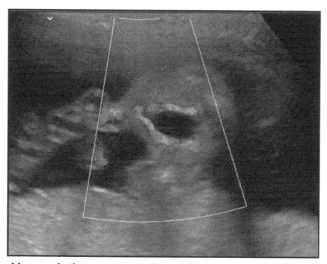

Normal three vessel cord: two arteries form a "V" around the bladder.

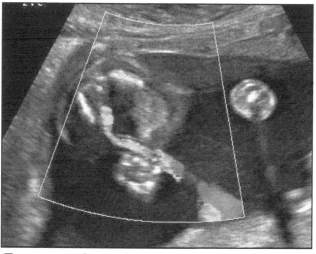

Two vessel cord: only one artery is noted along the side of the bladder.

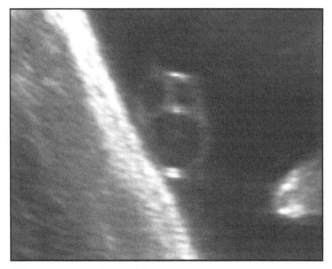

Three vessel cord in transverse

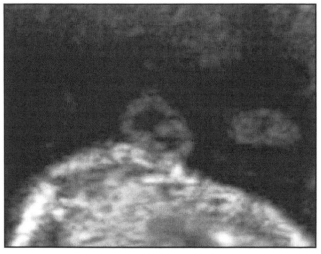

Two vessel cord in transverse

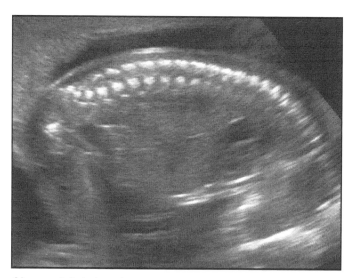

Normal fetal spine

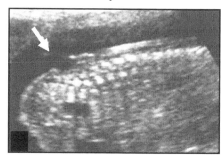

Spina bifida

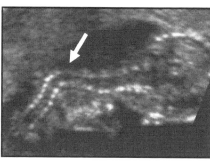

Scoliosis

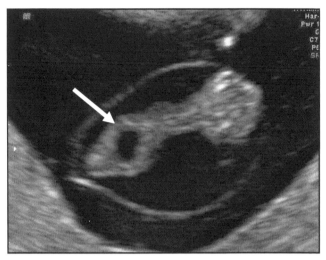

First trimester umbilical cord cyst

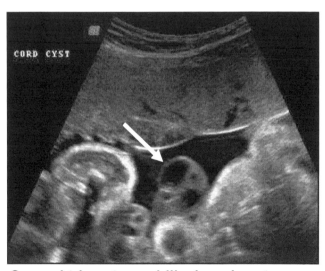

Second trimester umbilical cord cyst

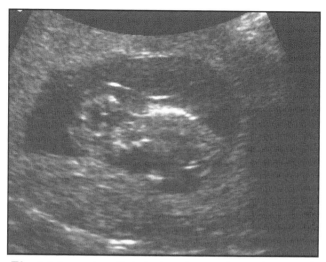

First trimester fetal demise: edema is noted around the fetus.

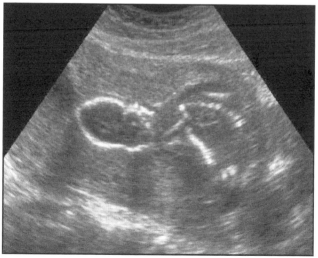

Second trimester fetal demise: the collapsing skull is known as the Spalding sign.

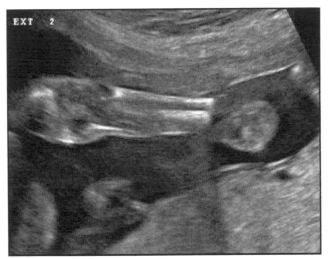

Normal lower extremity

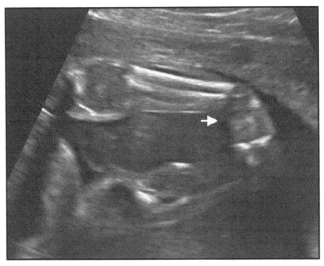

Club foot

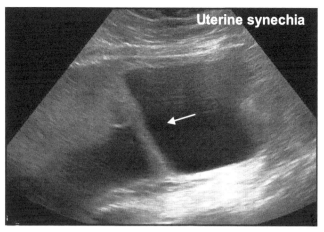

Uterine synechia and amniotic band: if you see an echogenic strip of tissue in the uterus, you need to determine if both ends are connected to the uterus or if one end is free-floating. A uterine synechia (above), or amniotic sheet, is a fibrous strip of uterine tissue and poses no harm to the fetus. An amniotic band (below) is sticky and can get tangled around fetal parts causing circulation to be cut off.

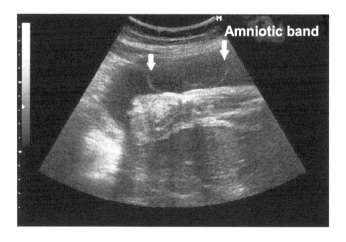

NOTES:

SONOGRAPHIC MARKERS OF COMMON FETAL SYNDROMES

- **Down's (Trisomy 21):** duodenal atresia, cardiac defects, cystic hygroma, thickened nuchal fold, omphalocele, short limbs, absent nasal bone, hyperechoic bowel, pyelectasis, ventriculomegaly, widened pelvic angle.
- **Edward's (Trisomy 13):** cardiac defects, IUGR, facial anomalies, cleft lip/palate, echogenic kidneys, rocker-bottom feet, encephalocele, spina bifida, pyelectasis, polydactyly, omphalocele, clubfoot, single umbilical artery, cystic hygroma.
- **Patau (Trisomy 18):** single umbilical artery, cardiac defects, clenched hands, club foot, choroid plexus cysts, enlarged cisterna magna, facial clefts, micrognathia, spina bifida, omphalocele, diaphragmatic hernia, kidney anomalies, polydactyly, hypotelorism, holoprosencephaly.
- **Beckwith-Wiedemann:** macrosomia, macroglossia, large kidneys, omphalocele.
- **Ivemark's:** polysplenia or asplenia, malpositioned organs, cardiac defects.
- **VATERS:** **V**ertebral anomalies/**V**entricular septal defects, **A**nal atresia, **T**racheo **E**sophageal fistula, **R**adial dysplasia/**R**enal abnormalities, **S**ingle umbilical artery.
- **Achondroplasia:** heterozygous type is non-lethal and includes limb shortening and mild macrocephaly; homozygous type is lethal and includes severe limb shortening, severe macrocephaly, narrow thorax.

- **Triploidy (three of every chromosome):** IUGR, hydrocephalus, oligohydramnios, syndactyly, macrocephaly, abnormally large or small placenta.
- **Meckel-Gruber:** autosomal recessive, polydactyly, encephalocele, polycystic kidneys.
- **Limb-body wall complex:** chorionic cavity and peritoneal cavity do not separate; umbilical cord and abdominal contents are trapped in between; limb defects, body wall defects, scoliosis.
- **Turner's:** cystic hygroma, cardiac anomalies, urinary tract anomalies.

THE FETAL HEART

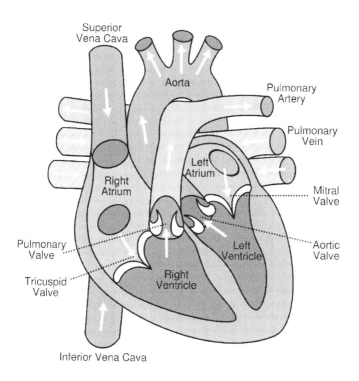

Superior Vena Cava

Aorta

Pulmonary Artery

Pulmonary Vein

Left Atrium

Mitral Valve

Right Atrium

Pulmonary Valve

Aortic Valve

Tricuspid Valve

Left Ventricle

Right Ventricle

Inferior Vena Cava

KEY POINTS FOR
THE FETAL HEART

By angling cephalad (toward the head) from a transverse view of the abdomen, you will see the 4 chamber view of the heart. The ventricles should be of similar size and the atria should be of similar size. Three hearts should be able to fit in the chest.

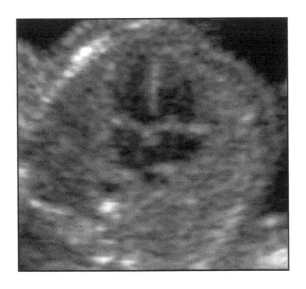

The mitral valve is between the LA and LV. The tricuspid valve is between the RA and the RV. Remember: "TRI to get it RIGHT".

From the 4 chamber view, angle further cephalad to see the left ventricle and the aorta (left ventricular outflow tract) in the same view.

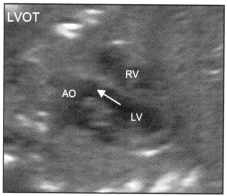

From the LVOT view, angle the probe further towards the head and slightly towards the fetal left shoulder. Here you will see the right ventricular outflow tract.

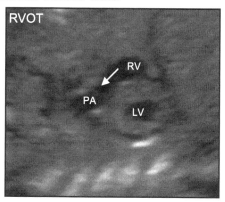

Be sure the outflow tracts cross each other in order to rule out transposition of the great vessels (pulmonary artery and aorta).

When evaluating the septum, the ultrasound beam should be perpendicular to the septum. If VSD (ventricular septal defect) is suspected, put color Doppler on and watch to see if color passes between the ventricles.

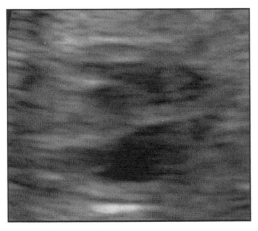

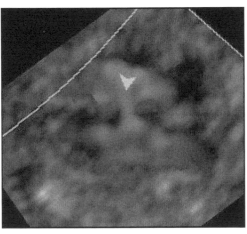

It is common to see an echogenic foci in the left ventricle. The fetus is at a slightly higher risk for Down's syndrome, but is usually normal if it is an isolated finding. *"Echogenic foci noted in the left ventricle."*

If you are listening to the fetal heart beat and you suspect an arythmia, watch the chest to be sure the fetus is not hiccupping.

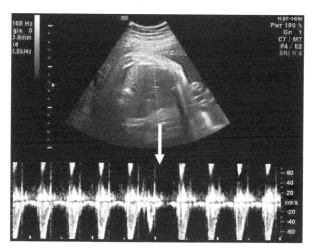

At this point, you won't be expected to identify all the different types of heart defects. Practice perfecting your four chamber and outflow tract images. When something doesn't look right, you'll know it.

MULTIPLES

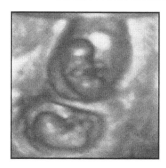
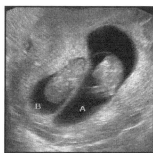
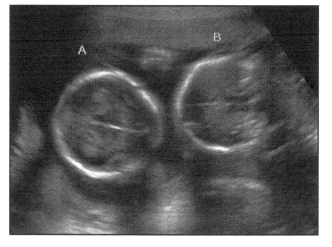

KEY POINTS FOR MULTIPLES:

🗝️ The fetus closest to the cervix at the initial scan is named Baby A. Never change the names of the babies because they have changed position. It is important to keep their names constant in order to track their growth.

🗝️ When initially scanning twins, finding the membrane will be the first clue to choronicity. If the wall/membrane interface looks like a tent (twin peak sign) this means they are dichorionic. If no peak is seen, they are monochorionic:

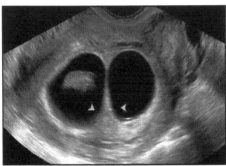

Dichorionic: twin peak sign has a tent appearance.

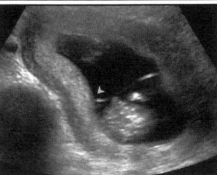

Monochorionic: no twin peak sign is seen at the membrane/ placenta interface.

There should be a < 20% difference between the fetal weights. To find the intertwin discordance (difference), take the largest weight minus the smaller weight, then divide that by the largest weight.

Twin A = 345 g   569
Twin B = 569 g   -345
                         224

$224 \div 569 = .39367 =$ **39% discordance**

	Monochorionic Monoamniotic	Monochorionic Diamniotic	Dichorionic Diamniotic
identical/ fraternal	identical	identical	monozygotic=identical dizygotic=fraternal
chorionic sacs	1	1	2
amniotic sacs	1	2	2
placentas	1	1	2
yolk sacs	1	2	2
membrane	none	thin membrane	thick/twin peak sign
gender	same	same	same or different

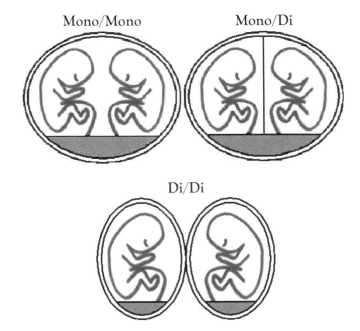

Mono/Mono   Mono/Di

Di/Di

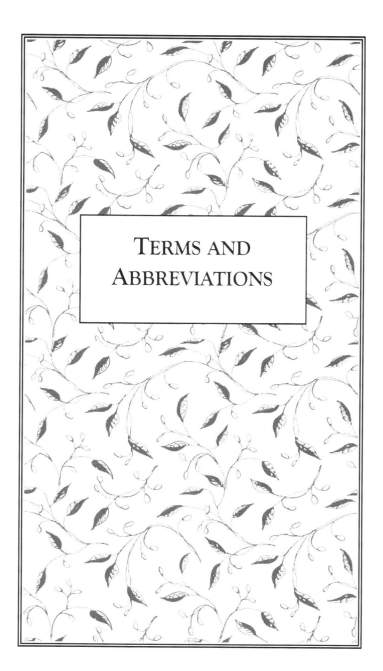

TERMS AND ABBREVIATIONS

acrania: having no skull above the eyes; leads to anencephaly.

adenomyosis: when endometrial tissue invades the muscular walls of the uterus.

AFP (alpha-fetoprotein): protein produced by the fetus, excreted into amniotic fluid and can be measured in maternal blood; high levels may indicate an open neural tube defect or other chromosomal disorder.

amenorrhea: absence of periods.

amniocentesis: a test to evaluate the chromosomes of the fetus.

amniotic fluid: the fluid that surrounds the fetus, produced by the placenta in early pregnancy, then produced by the fetal kidneys in later pregnancy.

amniotic sac: a thin-walled sac containing amniotic fluid that surrounds the fetus during pregnancy.

anencephaly: a condition where the fetus has minimal brain tissue due to being exposed to amniotic fluid.

anhydramnios: absence of amniotic fluid.

aqueductal stenosis: blockage of cerebral spinal fluid flow through the aqueduct of Sylvius (narrow canal through the center of the brain).

ARPKD (autosomal recessive polycystic kidney disease): enlarged, hyperechoic fetal kidneys.

atresia: congenital absence or closure of a body opening or tubular structure.

bowel herniation: a condition in which the fetal bowel herniates through a defect in the abdominal wall into the umbilical cord.

BTB (break through bleeding): bleeding between periods.

BSO (bilateral salpingo-oophorectomy): surgical removal of both fallopian tubes and ovaries.

BTL (bilateral tubal ligation): surgical procedure for sterilization; fallopian tubes are blocked and sealed.

CA-125: blood test used as an ovarian cancer marker, usually ordered after a suspicious ovarian mass is observed on ultrasound. <35 U/mL is considered normal.

cerclage: a stitch placed around the cervix to hold it closed as pregnancy advances.

Chiari malformation: a malformation of the posterior fossa of the brain where the brain and spinal cord connect.

corpus luteal cyst: cyst formed at the site of ovulation.

CRL (crown rump length): measurement of the fetus in the first trimester.

CVS (chorionic villus sampling): a procedure involving the removal of a small amount of placental tissue.

cystic teratoma (dermoid cyst): may contain hair, fat, bone or teeth; almost always benign; usually appears as an echogenic mass with cystic areas.

DUB (dysfunctional uterine bleeding): abnormal bleeding due to changes in hormone levels.

dysmenorrhea: painful periods.

dyspareunia: pain with sex.

eccentric cord insertion: cord inserted towards the side of the placenta.

echocardiogram: a specialized ultrasound that examines fetal heart structures and function.

EFW (estimated fetal weight): weight of the fetus; obtained by measuring the HC, BPD, AC and FL.

embryo: second through eighth week of prenatal development.

endometrioma: chocolate cyst, formed when endometriosis invades the ovary.

endometriosis: when endometrial tissue grows outside the uterus; not seen on ultrasound.

ERT: estrogen replacement therapy.

f-BhCG (free beta human chorionic gonadotropin): measures the amount of hCG in the maternal blood.

fetal fibronectin (FFN): a protein that glues the amniotic sac to the lining of the uterus. The presence of the protein in the maternal cervix may indicate the onset of labor.

fetal hydrops (aka hydrops fetalis): a life-threatening condition in which fluid accumulates in fetal tissues.

fetal surveillance testing: includes the biophysical profile, Doppler ultrasound of the umbilical cord and middle cerebral artery, and non-stress test.

fetus: eighth through fortieth weeks of prenatal development.

fibroid (leiomyoma): a non-cancerous growth of the uterus.

gastroschesis: fetal intestine protrudes through a defect adjacent to the cord insertion; it is not covered with a membrane and is not usually associated with chromosomal anomalies.

GDM (gestational diabetes mellitus): a condition that can develop during pregnancy when the body can't make enough insulin.

gravida: the number of times the mother has been pregnant, including a current pregnancy.

GS (gestational sac): seen on ultrasound at around 5 weeks gestation.

glucose screen: The glucose screen is used to check for diabetes at 24 weeks gestation.

hCG (human chorionic gonadotropin) test: A *qualitative* hCG test detects the presence or absence of hCG in the blood or urine (positive or negative result). A *quantitative* hCG test (or beta hCG) measures the amount of hCG actually present in the maternal blood.

hemorrhagic corpus luteal cyst: when bleeding occurs inside the corpus luteal cyst; may be described as having a "ground-glass" or spiderweb-like appearance.

hernia: an opening in the abdominal muscle through which a portion of intestine or other internal organ may protrude.

HRT: hormone replacement therapy.

HTN (hypertension): high blood pressure, may be chronic or gestational.

hydrocephalus: a buildup of cerebral spinal fluid causing pressure inside the head and the skull bones to expand.

hydronephrosis: dilatation in the fetal renal calyces.

hydrops fetalis (aka fetal hydrops): a life-threatening condition in which fluid accumulates in fetal tissues.

hydrosalpinx: fluid-filled fallopian tube; no flow seen with color Doppler.

hyperemesis: a complication of pregnancy characterized by nausea, vomiting, and dehydration.

hypoxia: decreased oxygen supply to the body's tissues.

hysterectomy: removal of the uterus and cervix (total), or removal of UT only (partial).

IUD (intrauterine device): metal or plastic device placed in the uterus for birth control or to control abnormal uterine bleeding; will appear as a bright linear echo within the endometrium.

IUGR (intrauterine growth restriction): when the EFW measures <10%.

IUP (intrauterine pregnancy): pregnancy in the uterus, as opposed to an ectopic.

keyhole bladder: a keyhole-like appearance of the fetal bladder seen on ultrasound that is characteristic of lower urinary tract obstruction due to posterior urethral valves; seen only in males.

LBW (low birth weight): infant with a birth weight of less than 2500 g (5 lb 8 oz), regardless of gestational age at the time of birth.

LGA (large for gestational age): when the fetus is gaining weight too rapidly; >90% EFW.

LH/FSH ratio (luteinizing hormone/follicle-stimulating hormone): abnormal ratio is a sign of PCOS.

LSO (left salpingo-oophorectomy): surgical removal of the left ovary.

MCDK (multicystic dysplastic kidney): multiple renal cysts of varying sizes that do not communicate.

menorrhagia: an abnormally heavy and prolonged menstrual period.

methotrexate: a drug used to treat an ectopic pregnancy.

metrorrhagia: uterine bleeding at irregular intervals.

MSAFP (maternal serum alpha-fetoprotein): performed between weeks 15 and 20 to determine the amount of AFP; level should be < 2.5 MoM (multiples of the median); increased MSAFP could indicate a fetal open neural tube defect; other reasons unrelated to the fetus include placental abnormalities, maternal ovarian or hepatic tumors.

MSD (mean sac diameter): average measurement of the gestational sac used to date a first trimester pregnancy prior to visualizing a fetal pole; add the length, width and height of the GS, then divide by three.

multiparous: having had two or more pregnancies.

nulliparous: having never been pregnant.

oligohydramnios: amniotic fluid volume under 5 cm.

omphalocele: fetal intestine, liver or both protrude through the base of the umbilical cord and are covered with a membrane; may be associated with chromosomal anomalies.

PAPP-A (pregnancy associated plasma protein A): a protein used in screening tests for Down syndrome.

para: the number of >20 weeks births (alive or stillborn); twins or triplets are still counted only as one birth.

PCOS (polycystic ovarian syndrome): ultrasonic appearance includes multiple subcentimeter follicles around the perimeter of the ovaries; may have abnormal FSH/LH ratio; most common symptoms are irregular periods, weight gain, excessive hair growth and acne.

PID (pelvic inflammatory disease): inflammation of the female genital tract, accompanied by fever and lower abdominal pain.

polyhydramnios: amniotic fluid volume over 25 cm.

polyp: a mass in the endometrium or cervix; may be flat or attached by a vascular stalk; most common symptom is irregular bleeding.

posterior urethral valves: an abnormality in which the urethra forms valves that partially or completely block urine outflow.

preeclampsia: when a pregnant woman develops high blood pressure and protein in the urine after the 20th week of pregnancy.

preterm: delivery before 37 weeks gestation.

PROM (premature rupture of membranes): rupture of the membrane of the amniotic sac and chorion more than one hour before the onset of labor.

pyelectasis: dilatation in the fetal renal pelvis.

retroplacental hematoma: bleeding contained behind the placenta.

Rh Antibody: If the mother is Rh negative, her blood will be tested during the sixth or seventh month to see if there is an antibody being produced that might harm the baby's blood. If there is none, then she will be given a shot to prevent the antibody from being formed.

RPOC (retained products of conception): placental and/or fetal tissue that remains in the uterus after a spontaneous pregnancy loss (miscarriage), planned pregnancy termination, or term delivery.

RSO (right salpingo-oophorectomy): surgical removal of the right ovary.

salpingo-oophorectomy: removal of the ovary and fallopian tube.

SGA (small for gestational age): babies that are below the 10th percentile in weight for the gestational age.

stuck twin: the donor twin in twin-to-twin transfusion syndrome; twin appears to be stuck to the wall of the uterus due to severe oligohydramnios.

SUA (single umbilical artery): fetus with one umbilical artery as opposed to the normal two umbilical arteries.

subamniotic hematoma: the pooling of blood between the amnion and chorion.

subchorionic hematoma: the pooling of blood between the chorion and the uterine wall.

TAH (total abdominal hysterectomy): surgical removal of the uterus and the cervix.

TOLAC (trial of labor after cesarean): patient may be allowed to labor on her own for a vaginal delivery after a previous c-section.

TTTS (twin-to-twin transfusion syndrome): a condition in identical twins with a shared placenta that contains connections between the twins blood vessels. The donor twin will be smaller with little amniotic fluid; the recipient twin will be larger with too much amniotic fluid.

VBAC (vaginal birth after cesarean): the practice of birthing a baby vaginally after a previous baby has been delivered through caesarean section.

velamentous cord: cord inserted directly into the amnion, as opposed to the placenta.

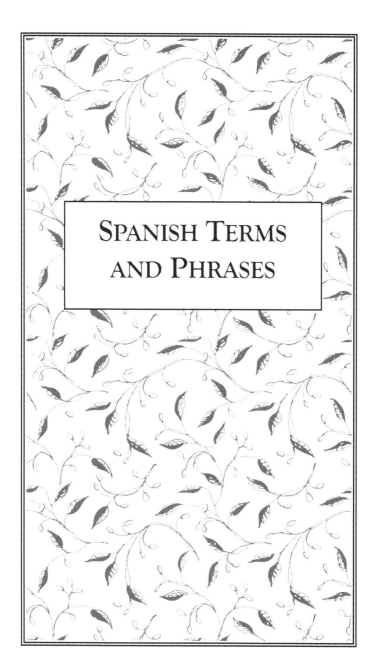

SPANISH TERMS
AND PHRASES

- Head = cabeza
- Eyes = ojos
- Nose = nariz
- Mouth = boca
- Lips = labios
- Ear = oido
- Hair = pelo
- Hand = mano
- Foot = pie
- Fingers = dedos
- Toes = dedos de pie
- Abdomen = abdomen
- Bladder = vejiga
- Stomach = estómago
- Arm = brazo
- Leg = pierna
- Heart = corazón
- Femur = el fémur
- Skull = el cráneo
- Spine = la vertebra

- Ovaries = ovarios
- Uterus = útero
- Cervix = cuello del tero
- Penis = el pene
- Scrotum = el escroto
- Vagina = la vagina
- Hot = calor
- Warm = caliente
- Cold = frío
- Polyp = el pólipo
- Hysterectomy = la histerectomia
- Ultrasound = la sonografia
- Contractions = las contracciones
- Yes = Sí
- No = No

- Left = izquierdo
- Right = derecho
- He = el
- Is = es
- I = me
- You = tu
- She = ella
- They = ellos
- Us/we= nosotras
- Like = gusta
- And = y
- Or = o

- But = pero
- If = si
- Because = porque
- It is = esta
- Where = donde
- Where is = donde est
- How = cómo
- When = cuando
- Who = quien
- What = que
- Why = por qué
- Here = aquí

Numbers:

1. Uno
2. Dos
3. Tres
4. Cuatro
5. Cinco
6. Seis
7. Siete
8. Ocho
9. Nueve
10. Diez
11. Once
12. Doce
13. Trece
14. Catorce
15. Quince
16. Dieciséis
17. Diecisiete
18. Dieciocho
19. Diecinueve
20. Veinte
21. Veintiuno
22. Veintidós
23. Veintitrés
24. Veinticuatro
25. Veinticinco
26. Veintiséis
27. Veintisiete
28. Veintiocho
29. Veintinueve
30. Treinta
31. Treinta y uno

Dates:

- January: enero
- February: febrero
- March: marzo
- April: abril
- May: mayo
- June: junio
- July: julio
- August: agosto
- September: septiembre
- October: octubre
- November: noviembre
- December: diciembre

- Tomorrow: mañana
- Today is: Hoy es ___.

- Monday: lunes
- Tuesday: martes
- Wednesday: miércoles
- Thursday: jueves
- Friday: viernes
- Saturday: sabádo
- Sunday: domingo

- Good morning: *Buenos días.*
- Good afternoon: *Buenas tardes.*
- My name is ____: *Me llamo_____.*
- I am the sonographer: *Yo soy la sonografista.*
- I speak very little Spanish: *Yo hablo muy poco español.*
- I don't understand: *No entiendo.*
- What is your name? *¿Cómo se llama usted?*
- What is your date of birth? *¿Cuál es su fecha de nacimiento?*
- Social security number? *¿Número de seguro social?*
- How are you? *¿Cómo esta usted?*
- Fine thank you. And you? *Bien, gracias. ¿Y usted?*
- Good, well: *bien, bueno*
- Okay: *regular*
- Sick: *enfermo*
- Not well: *mal*
- Better: *mejor*
- A little better: *un poco mejor*
- Tired: *cansado*
- Worse: *peor*
- What symptoms do you have? *¿Qué síntomas tiene?*
- Nausea: *náusea*
- Vomiting: *vómito*
- Dizziness: *mareo*
- Fatigue: *fatiga*
- Headache: *dolor de cabeza*
- Do you have pain? *¿Tiene dolor?*
- Where is the pain? *¿Dónde está el dolor?* or *¿Dónde te duele?*
- When was your last period? *¿Cuándo comenzo su último periodo?*
- Are your periods regular? *¿Sus períodos son regulares?*

- Have you had any cramping or bleeding? *¿Ha tenido usted algun dolor o sangrado?*
- Are you bleeding? *¿Sangrado?*
- How long have you had (bleeding, pain)? *¿Cuánto tiempo___?*
- It has been (two) days: *Hace dos días.*
- How long does the pain last: *¿Cuánto tiempo dura el dolor?*
- Since this morning: *desde esta mañana*
- Last night: *anoche*
- Yesterday: *ayer*
- Last week: *semana pasada*
- Do you have hypertension? *¿Tiene presión alta?*
- Do you have diabetes/GDM? *¿Tiene diabetes?*
- Are you allergic to latex? *¿Tiene alérgia al latex?*
- Are you allergic to betadine? *¿Tiene alérgia al iodo?*
- This is a transvaginal exam: *Este es un examen transvaginal.*
- Please go the the restroom and empty your bladder: *Por favor vaya al baño y orine.*
- Please undress from the waist down: *Por favor desnudese de la cintura para abajo.*
- Please cover with this paper drape: *Por favor cubrese con este ropage.*
- Please lie down on the table: *Por favor acuéstese en la mesa.*
- Place your feet here: *Ponga sus pies aqui.*
- Scoot down to the end of the table: *Baje hasta el borde de la mesa.*
- It is a boy: *Es un niño.*
- It is a girl: *Es une niña.*

- I am going to measure the baby: *Voy a medir el bebe.*
- The baby weighs _pounds, _ounces: *El/La bebé pesa _libra, _onzas.*
- Now you can get dressed: *Ahora se puede vestir.*
- The doctor will give you the results: *El doctor le dará los resultados.*
- Please have a seat in the waiting room: *Por favor sientese en la sala de espera.*

NOTES:

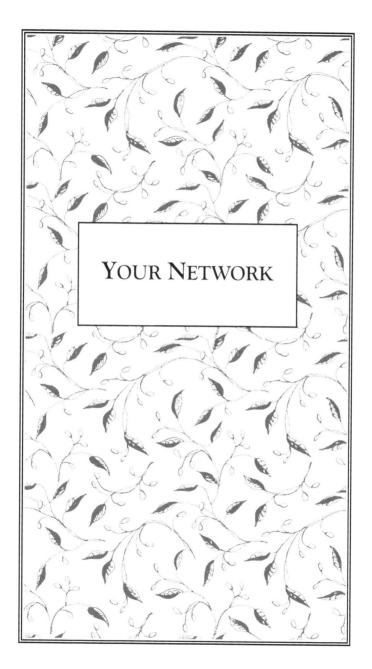

YOUR NETWORK

NAME/SITE	PHONE #/EMAIL

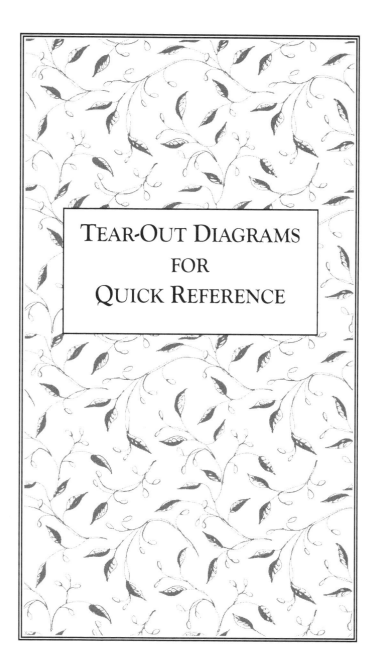

TEAR-OUT DIAGRAMS
FOR
QUICK REFERENCE

UTERUS	FUNDAL CONTOUR	INNER CONTOUR AND CAVITY
Normal	convex	straight across or convex
Arcuate	convex or mildly concave	indented <1.5 cm
Bicornuate	concave	indented partially or completely to the cervix
Septate	convex	septated completely to the cervix
Subseptate	convex	septated > 1.5 cm

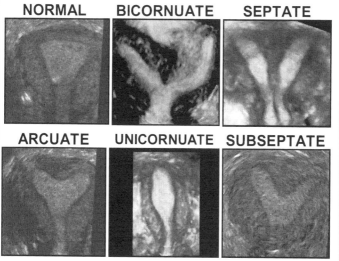

NORMAL   **BICORNUATE**   **SEPTATE**

ARCUATE   **UNICORNUATE**   **SUBSEPTATE**

GS cm	Wks/Days	CRL cm
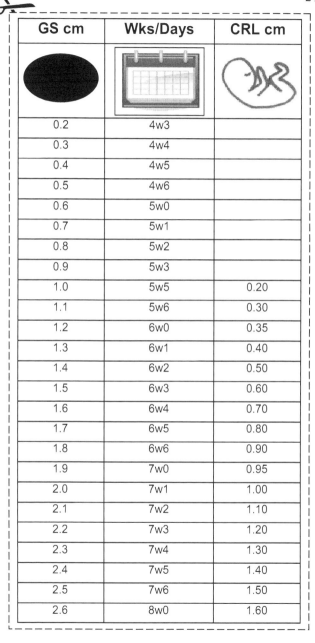		
0.2	4w3	
0.3	4w4	
0.4	4w5	
0.5	4w6	
0.6	5w0	
0.7	5w1	
0.8	5w2	
0.9	5w3	
1.0	5w5	0.20
1.1	5w6	0.30
1.2	6w0	0.35
1.3	6w1	0.40
1.4	6w2	0.50
1.5	6w3	0.60
1.6	6w4	0.70
1.7	6w5	0.80
1.8	6w6	0.90
1.9	7w0	0.95
2.0	7w1	1.00
2.1	7w2	1.10
2.2	7w3	1.20
2.3	7w4	1.30
2.4	7w5	1.40
2.5	7w6	1.50
2.6	8w0	1.60

GA Weeks	Length in inches	Size of a:
8	1.5	raspberry
10	2.4	prune
12	3.5	plum
14	4.7	lemon
16	6.25	avocado
18	7.8	sweet potato
20	9.75	banana
22	11	papaya
24	11.7	cantaloupe
26	12.5	lettuce
28	13.65	eggplant
30	14.8	cucumber
32	15.6	squash
34	16.4	butternut squash
36	17.5	coconut
38	18.7	honeydew
40	19.5	watermelon

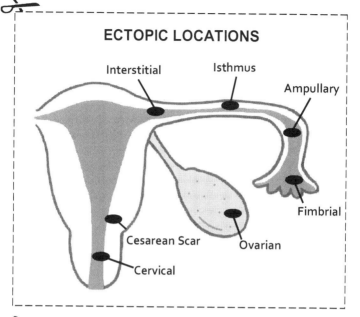

ECTOPIC LOCATIONS

Interstitial

Isthmus

Ampullary

Fimbrial

Cesarean Scar

Ovarian

Cervical

First Trimester Measurements:

- Gestational sac:
    visualized at about 5 weeks (800-2000 IU hCg)

- Yolk sac:
    visualized at about 5.5 weeks (2000 IU hCg)
    GS msd = 8 mm; YS should measure < 6 mm

- Embryo:
    visualized between 5.5-6.0 weeks
    GS msd = 16 mm

- Cardiac activity:
    visualized when CRL = 5 mm
    (about 5.5–6.0 weeks)

	Monochorionic Monoamniotic	Monochorionic Diamniotic	Dichorionic Diamniotic
identical/fraternal	identical	identical	monozygotic=identical dizygotic=fraternal
fetuses	2	2	2
chorionic sacs	1	1	2
amniotic sacs	1	2	2
placentas	1	1	2
yolk sacs	1	2	2
membrane	none	thin membrane	thick/twin peak sign
gender	same	same	same or different

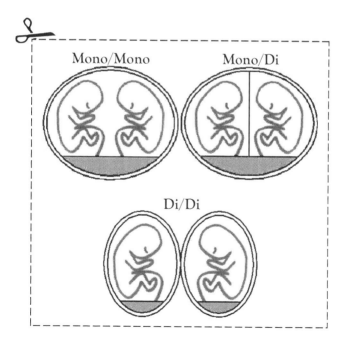

Mono/Mono   Mono/Di

Di/Di

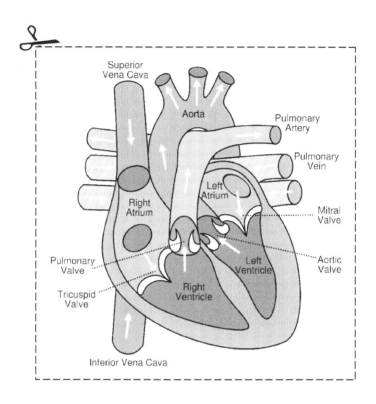

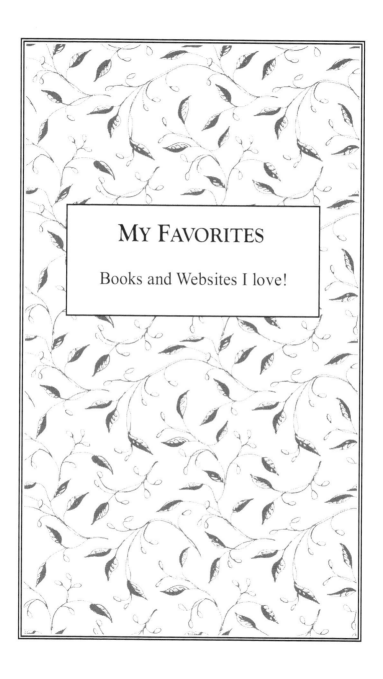

My Favorites

Books and Websites I love!

Books:

These are some of the ultrasound books I like to keep close at hand:

- <u>Step by Step: Ultrasound in Gynecology</u>
  by Kuldeep Singh, MD & Narendra Malhotra, MD
  -this book comes with a photo cd-rom; it has great explanations of gynecological findings, as well as full color pictures. Also a nice, small size.

- <u>Diagnostic Imaging: Obstetrics</u>
  by Paula Woodward, MD
  -I had the great fortune of meeting Dr. Woodward at the AIUM conference in Orlando, FL. She is a wonderful teacher who made the presentation so interesting! I love this book because, although it is a large textbook style book, it is written in bullet-point format, so it's really easy to follow.

- <u>Structural Fetal Abnormalities</u>
  by Roger C. Sanders
  -very comprehensive, lots of images and sonographic markers, plus recommended obstetrical management (good to know how the doctor will handle this type of patient.)

Websites:

www.ARDMS.org

www.SDMS.org

www.ob-ultrasound.net

www.radiopaedia.org

www.brooksidepress.org

www.sonoguide.com

www.fetal.com/

www.med.upenn.edu/fetus/echo.htm

www.ultrasoundcases.info/category.aspx?cat=65

www.ultrasound-images.com—ob and gyn

http://radiology.rsna.org/content/254/2/342.figures-only

www.diagnosticimaging.com

123sonography.com

http://www.fetalmedicineusa.com (click online education)

www.ultrasoundpaedia.com

SOURCES

Ultrasound Images reproduced with permission from:
Women's Care Florida, Ob & Gyn Specialists and
Dr. Beryl R. Benacerraf

Diagrams and graphics:
Dr. Frank Gaillard, Dr. Michael Hughey and
Rebecca S. Willis, copyright 2013
Fetal heart diagram: https://en.wikipedia.org/wiki/
File:Diagram_of_the_human_heart_(cropped).svg

Woodward, Paula, et al. *Diagnostic Imaging: Obstetrics*, Amirsys/
Elsevier Saunders, 2005. Print

Callen, Peter. *Ultrasonography in Obstetrics and Gynecology*.
Philadelphia: W.B. Saunders Company, 1994. Print

Lin, Edward P, et al. "Diagnostic Clues to Ectopic Pregnancy."
Radiographics.rsna.org, 2008. Web

Jaffe, Richard and Jacques S. Abramowics, *Manual of Obstetric
and Gynecologic Ultrasound.* Philadelphia: Lippincott Raven,
1997. Print

Stanislarsky, Alexandra and Frank Gaillard. "Uterine
Anatomical Abnormalities," *Radiopaedia.org.* Web, July 2013

"Why is it important to diagnose chorionicity and how do we
do it?" *Best Practice & Research, Clinical Obstetrics and
Gynaecology* 2004, Print, 4:515-530.

Cuillier, Fabrice, Eva Racanska, Philippe Jeanty. "Uterine Scar
Dehiscence," *thefetus.net* 2010, Web February 2013

Henningsen, Charlotte, "Cervical Incompetence: Sonography Techniques and Pitfalls," SDMS lecture 2013

Foy, Pamela M., "Cervical Sonography Technique," Ohio State University Medical Center; Lecture via web

Bermejo, Carmina, et al. "Three Dimensional Ultrasonography in the Diagnosis of Mullerian Duct Anomalies," Donald School Journal of Ultrasound in Obstetrics and Gynecology, January-March 2009; 3(1): 21-30, Web

Nardozza, L.M., et al. "Prenatal Diagnosis of Amniotic Band Syndrome in the Third Trimester of Pregnancy using 3D Ultrasound." Clinical Imaging Science, June 2013. Web

Rajanna, D.K., et al. "Autosomal Recessive Polycystic Kidney Disease: Antenatal Diagnosis and Histopathological Correlation." Clinical Imaging Science, June 2013. Web

Nyberg, David A., Souter, Vivienne L., "Sonographic Markers of Fetal Trisomies, Second Trimester," 2001 American Institute of Ultrasound in Medicine. Web

Made in the USA
Las Vegas, NV
06 August 2022

52807691R00133